"I loved every page of this book: funny, sad, romantic, and full of pigeons—glorious but underappreciated, mysterious yet near at hand, each an individual, their dramas unseen right under our noses. Yet for Buckbee, suffering from a broken heart and broken body, birds like the injured Two-Step fling open doors of enchantment, healing, and communion. He's right: We really *should* all be birds—but since we can't, the best remedy I can think of is this book."

—Sy Montgomery,
author of *Of Time and Turtles:
Mending the World, Shell by Shattered Shell*

"*We Should All Be Birds* is a beautifully intimate memoir about relentless love despite unrelenting pain. It's compulsively readable and unexpectedly reassuring in times that seem to have lost their footing. And yes, the birds are the real medicine. Especially one particular, peculiar little one."

—Carl Safina,
author of *Alfie and Me:
What Owls Know, What Humans Believe*

"At once painful and joyful, *We Should All Be Birds* is an immersive tale of chronic life, in which a bird allows a man to love him, which allows the author to finally love himself. Even in pain."

—Richard Louv,
author of *Our Wild Calling:
How Connecting with Animals Can
Transform Our Lives—and Save Theirs*

"Brian Buckbee has discovered a slower, more open-hearted, humble stance toward living and creating, where small joy is in no way insubstantial, and where attention given freely—to the birds he cares for who ultimately care for him, and to the needs of body and spirit—creates unexpected forms of love and devotion."

—Lia Purpura,
author of *All the Fierce Tethers*

"Brian Buckbee has sent us a series of gentle, funny, poignant, honest, and loving messages-in-a-bottle from the country of long-term illness and cross-species friendship. Reading *We Should All Be Birds* feels like stumbling into the serendipity of a conversation with a stranger that leaves you changed. With sweet lyricism, it accompanies you from darkness into connection. This story of a man's friendship with a pigeon serves as a reminder that living beyond yourself, entwined with the lives of other creatures, can save you when the human world fails to. It is a gift to spend time with Buckbee and his companion Two-Step."

—Eiren Caffall,
author of *The Mourner's Bestiary*

We Should All Be Birds

We Should All Be Birds

(a memoir)

Brian Buckbee

with CAROL ANN FITZGERALD

TIN HOUSE
PORTLAND, OREGON

Copyright © 2025 Brian Buckbee and Carol Ann Fitzgerald

First US Edition 2025
Printed in the United States of America

Manufacturing by Lake Book Manufacturing
Interior design by Beth Steidle

Library of Congress Cataloging-in-Publication Data is available.

Tin House
2617 NW Thurman Street, Portland, OR 97210
www.tinhouse.com

Distributed by W. W. Norton & Company

1 2 3 4 5 6 7 8 9 0

Contents

We Should All Be Birds

Part 1

(JANUARY 2022)

MY RESCUE PIGEON AND I FOUND EACH OTHER AT THE very beginning of the pandemic, when we were both dealing with crippling health problems. As time went on, he got better. As time went on, I got worse.

I am lying in bed, saying these words in the dark, hoping that tomorrow I can dictate all that I remember to my computer. My migraine has reached epic proportions. It helps to think about my pigeon (Two-Step) and his new girlfriend (V.) in the living room in the little nest I helped them make high up on a shelf. At night, when I try to fall asleep to escape the headache that never goes away (the headache that makes it impossible for me to read and write), I can hear Two-Step making soft *chukking* sounds. I think it may be his way of telling a story to V. to help her fall back to sleep.

It is hard to admit, but they are not the only pigeons flying at large in my house. I've taken in other wounded birds, all pigeons except for a ring-necked dove, and with their offspring, there are enough to fill a table at the Last Supper. In the morning, when my headache wakes me, I open my bedroom door, and all the birds take flight. Feathers fly. Some of the babies poke their heads above the rim of the baskets their parents have built nests in. I quickly find my corner of the couch, plop down, stretch my legs out on the coffee table, pull down over my eyes the soft beanie that the woman I loved knit for me a long time ago, and begin to do the math that helps me figure out how many hours I need to get through before night comes and I can find solace in sleep.

These wild pigeons are in my house because it is against the law for the bird rehabilitator to rescue them. "Pigeons are considered an invasive species," she told me over the phone. Apparently, if I brought a wounded eagle, hummingbird, or vulture to her, she could have taken it in, but a sick baby starling or a fluffy little house sparrow she would have to turn away. This was just after I found Two-Step, who was malnourished and had a deformed leg that prevented him from walking properly, and I had no idea that he was going to save my life.

———

YOU MAY NOT BE CRAZY about pigeons. I understand—I lived in a city once. But pigeons never "invaded" anything. We snatched them out of the wild and held them captive. This was ten thousand or so years ago. We domesticated them because we liked to eat them, and use their feathers for decoration, and sacrifice them by the thousands so the gods would stop treating us so bad.

———

I MET TWO-STEP on May 14, 2020, on a warm spring night when the green foliage was bursting forth like a miracle. Now, as I tell myself these words, propped up in bed with the lights off, a winter storm shaking the windowpane beside me, it is hard to believe our meet-cute happened almost two years ago.

It was my habit back then to go for a stroll around my residential neighborhood every evening to distract myself from the black monster. The black monster was what I called my headache. My neurologist had different language—"migraine," "intractable headache," "new persistent daily headache"—terms that were interchangeable and always fell short of the mark. I had been visited by the monster for the first time on the night of March 19 the previous year, and this meant that on the day I met Two-Step for the first time, I'd had a headache for 422 days straight. The headache was the most disastrous symptom of the mystery illness that had overtaken me, but its other symptoms could also be intense—muscle weakness, shaking, seizures, nausea, and extensive body pain that followed even the smallest amounts of exertion.

My evening walks usually failed to reduce my pain, but they gave me some psychological relief, because I knew at the end of the walk I could crawl into bed and, when I fell asleep, I'd finally escape the monster.

The first two blocks of my evening walk were northbound (directions are important to me because, as a migraine sufferer, I need to be aware of the sun's position at all times). If you were a neighbor of mine, what you would have seen if you looked out your window was a person who was slumped over, shuffling his feet, baseball cap pulled down low. You would likely have thought I was a meth head. Or maybe you would have thought, "This guy is about to steal something"—and not something fancy like fine jewels or an entertainment center, but rather something pedestrian like a garden sprinkler or a chicken.

At the end of those two blocks, I'd turn left on the Kim Williams Trail. Kim Williams was a famous naturalist who lived a long time ago, but another Kim Williams was a very pretty-smelling girl I got to slow dance with in seventh grade while nervous sweat rolled down my back. (I'm guessing that Kim Williams has no memory of the brief dance we shared, swaying beneath the spinning disco ball at Daniel Wright Junior High School, but it is strangely consoling to me now that I have physical contact with no one at all.)

That one block west on the trail takes you to the Montana Natural History Center, and I knew from just looking through the windows that the building was full of all kinds of stuffed birds, birds that were enjoying their wild lives before some so-called sportsman or naturalist shot the shit out of them.

The western block of that walk was the most difficult for me *because* it faced west, and west meant sunset. Sunset is still one of the few headache triggers I experience. When that life-sustaining radiance stabs me in the eyes, it travels deep into my brain, where it plucks guitar strings attached to something deep down inside my gut.

At the end of that block, I'd reach Hickory Street and turn left, which faces south. But before I could turn south, I had to first confront the building directly across the street, a squat one-story office building that has always had particular significance to me. On the east side of the building was a newly erected metal-barred six-foot fence, about my height. There was a gap in the fence at the entrance to the parking lot, which had been recently paved and painted with bright-white parking-space lines. The grounds around this fancy building were neatly manicured, the grass lawn thick and neatly trimmed, and it was on the edge of that building's roof that I first saw Two-Step.

At that point, he was just an ordinary pigeon, though the way he was balancing on one leg made him look more like he thought he was a flamingo. He was staring at me, but I was afraid of catching a glimpse of the yellow torture ball (the sun) that would shoot flaming arrows into my eyeballs. So I turned onto Hickory Street and walked about a block. When I stopped to catch my breath, I was startled to see the same bird on the roof of the parked car next to me, looking me over with his golden eyes, once again while standing on one leg.

It was rare to see a pigeon in my neighborhood at that time, but it was even odder to see this particular pigeon standing so close that I could reach out and touch him. That first pandemic summer brought all sorts of unexpected animals into my neighborhood—bears and foxes, mountain lions, more deer than usual (including the one that birthed two fawns in my yard), and, on one particularly brilliant summer evening, a roly-poly, furry badger that scurried down Cottonwood Street, hugging the curb with so much exuberance he was applauded by people like me who were out watering their lawns. It seemed the farther we were forced away from people, the closer the animals got.

I stood still and looked at the bird who would become Two-Step. He appeared to want something from me, so I asked, "What do you want?" Talking to a bird may seem strange now, but for those of us who had been isolated from all humans by the pandemic, it was not unusual to go several days in a row without speaking at all. The sound of my voice surprised me, but it didn't surprise the bird, who just continued to contemplate me. When I decided to see how tame he was by reaching out to touch the plumage on his head, he awkwardly launched off from his one good leg and fluttered up to the railing of a nearby apartment porch.

I still had my headache, but the encounter gave me a small jolt of joy. This beautiful creature was curious about me! I walked another block south on Hickory, turned left on First Street, and soon was propped up in bed, eyes closed, my reliable plastic vomit bin on the floor, listening to the soothing voice of the PBS *Frontline* narrator, who lulled me to sleep while talking about how some part of the world was falling to pieces.

———

THE NEXT DAY was May 15, a special day on the calendar for me, as it is the birthday of my late mother.

My mother loved animals, and as a little boy, I rescued a bunch of injured birds with her. She'd lead me into our garage, where we kept them in cardboard boxes, and sometimes she'd open a box to show me a bird that had died, and I would cry and hug her legs before running up to my room to lie face down on my bed while waiting for her to come and comfort me, the way only a mother can. Sometimes the comfort from my mother came in the form of a glass of ginger ale with the perfect number of ice cubes, and sometimes the comfort was her tracing circles on my back while promising, "Everything is going to be okay."

My walk the next evening was the same as the previous day, except the pigeon wasn't on top of the office building, standing on his one leg at the very edge of the roof, teetering, like a desperate person thinking about stepping off into the abyss. The sky was filling with purples and reds, and the sadist golden-orb-king (the sun) was ready to dip beneath the railroad trestle and shoot his scorching light straight into my tender pupils.

The office building I mentioned earlier was not just any old office building. Besides being a sleekly designed chunk of modern architecture, located just three blocks from where I live, it also happened to house the therapist's office of the woman I loved. She—let's call her L.—was no longer in my life (she vanished one day and never came back), but we'd spent some mostly wonderful times on the couch, talking with her therapist about our future together, seeking advice on navigating the maelstrom of disapproval our relationship had elicited in our close-knit circle of friends.

Sometimes on my walks I would even see L.'s car in the parking lot, and I knew it was her car because there had been a time I had driven that car myself. The car would be parked between the bright-white lines on the jet-black asphalt, and I would gather that some mystery was going on inside the building that I would never know a thing about.

I once drove that car to meet L. after she found an abandoned gosling when she was jogging along a wooded nature path. This was in the spring of 2014. She called me to help her rescue the little goose and I hopped in the car and met her near the creek, which was high with spring runoff. L. went downstream while I tried to grab the little puffball, but he made his way into the rushing waters and began bobbing off, like a bath toy in a bubbling Jacuzzi, and he would have bobbed right past L. except she performed a miraculous feat and somehow swept him up in her jacket before he sped past her. I still tremble thinking about what would've happened to that puffball if she hadn't snagged him. What would have become of him downstream? He was just a handful of yellow down in the swollen, frothy waters of Rattlesnake Creek.

The bird rehabilitator—the same one who years later would teach me how to save Two-Step—told me and L. how to care for the gosling until we could do a soft release with him. A soft release basically means you get the bird healthy enough to return to his natural environment when he is ready. We were worried—he was so small, and he wasn't eating the Cheerios we put in a bowl for him. But the bird rehabilitator said, "Just float the cereal in some water," and that made all the difference, because as soon as we did that, the gosling started eating. To help a bird, what you really need to do is think like a bird.

Whereas Two-Step wanted to stand on my head after I found him, the baby goose wanted to nestle into my armpit. I think he thought I was a goose, my armpit the underside of his mother's wing, which was the best place to hide and stay warm and snuggle with his brothers and sisters. His squirming felt really good, and it kind of tickled, too. And when my armpit proved to be dissatisfying to him, probably because he realized I was no goose, he tried to wiggle his way into L.'s armpit, and then the two of us were giggling. A baby goose can create a lot of love in a tiny spare room that has nothing in it but a cardboard box, a heat lamp, and a bowl of Cheerios.

The next day L. and I released the gosling in a neighborhood pond, but the release was anything but soft. The bird rehabilitator had told us to put the baby goose in the water close to another goose family. She said it would find a place with the other babies and the parents would think of it as one of their own. But, for whatever reason, the first goose family we selected did *not* want our baby goose around *at all*. Our baby goose would paddle hopefully up to the family, and the parents would suddenly bare their sharp goose teeth and honk like cars on a busy highway and chase it away. At times our baby goose would basically be running on the water (impressive), and at other times he would dive beneath the water, his wings tucked in, swimming as fast as a yellow torpedo (even more impressive).

Then he'd surface and bob his way back toward the goose family and try again, and again he'd get chased away. For a while he floated alone in the middle of the pond, scared and exhausted. Maybe he sensed his fate was to be solo in the world, hanging on for as long as he could before a hawk or some other misfortune found him.

I was so pissed at those other geese that I decided to get back in the pond (I still had my waders on) and rescue the baby goose (again). I stomped and splashed after it, disturbing all sorts of wildlife, including flocks of birds that rocketed from the tall marsh grasses into the blue sky. And then an old guy walking along the path started yelling at me. He said he was calling the cops. I had spent the last nearly sleepless twenty-four hours with the woman I loved trying to save this little creature, and now my nerves were frayed and water was seeping into my cheap plastic waders and this grump who would probably kick a pigeon if it got too close to his penny-loafered foot was going to call the cops on me? The simple truth is (pardon the language) I was really in no mood to be fucked with. I think I may even have yelled something like "Go fuck yourself!" But to be fair, he was just trying to get a madman out of a pond and save the wild creatures from torment.

L. and I were not about to give up. That was our little goose! And lo, another miracle! A ray of light came shining through the clouds as L. caught the baby goose again.

We took him to the far side of the pond, where another goose family was sitting on the shore. As we approached, they waddled off into the water, and we placed the gosling in the shallows and he paddled straight ahead until he was perfectly aligned in the trail of goslings behind the parents. He was the last one in the line, but it was obvious he was welcome, and it was clear he belonged.

The following summer, after a very tough day, I went back to the pond to see if he was still there. I ended up sitting on the sloped bank not far from where the old guy had suggested I needed some kind of police intervention. I saw several clusters of geese cruise by, and though I couldn't tell for sure, I thought I spotted him. I tracked his progress across the pond for a while. "Hi, old friend," I said out loud. "You used to take comfort under my arm."

THE CONFUSION THAT COMES with my headache can be advantageous. When you are in the fog, you escape everything else. You can be with that little goose and the woman who saved it. You can feel a flat webbed foot on the palm of your hand and the long, loose hair of the woman you loved brushing against your cheek as you look up at the night sky.

ON MY SECOND evening walk, after I passed L.'s therapy building and didn't see the bird on top of it, I came to the swinging yellow gate in the middle of Hickory Street that is used on baseball game days to keep traffic (an invasive species) out of the neighborhood.

There on the post that anchored the gate was a pigeon, surely the same pigeon, standing on one leg, looking right at me. Was he following me? He had the funniest look in his eye, one of familiarity, as if we had known each other for a long, long time.

It was such a singular experience that, when mixed with my migraine-induced befuddlement, I began to think I was the subject of someone's elaborate prank.

I walked toward the bird, as I had the previous evening, but this time he didn't move. I stopped a couple of feet away from him and said something like, "You again?" He just stood there, as if about to speak. I wanted to stay longer, but I couldn't. I was about to get sick all over the street, and I hurried home as fast as I could and collapsed into bed.

———

WHEN I SAW the bird the third evening, something shifted in me.

He was on the roof of the therapy building again, and as I looked up at him looking down at me, I thought, "I have a role to play in your life."

I felt uneasy as I walked into the parking lot of the therapy building. After all, this was L.'s turf, and it felt like I was intruding. The lot was empty, the sun was setting (but safely behind the buildings of the new Sawmill District), and the air was getting cool. I knelt on the ground by the building and called the bird down. I think I said, "Come down, bird."

And he actually came down.

He had trouble flying, wobbling like a World War II plane attempting to land after being shot up in a dogfight, but he settled pretty close to me on the green grass, hopping around on his one good leg. He kept coming up close to me and then hopping away. He seemed to want something, and I figured what he wanted was food. Since there was not much daylight left, I rushed home, trying not to jostle my head and awaken the migraine monster. At home, I searched the cupboards, trying to find something that a pigeon might like to eat. I grabbed the last of my Club Crackers and raced back to where I'd left the bird and looked

Buckbee & Fitzgerald

around desperately for him. Had I missed my chance? I looked everywhere, but he was nowhere to be found. Maybe I hadn't run fast enough. Maybe I hadn't fully grasped the danger he was in. Whatever had happened to him . . . was clearly all my fault.

But then I spotted him! He was up on the roof of the therapy building. He hopped to the edge, swooped down, and landed by my feet. I knelt down, crumbled up some crackers, and spread them on the grass. And he ate.

I had learned from my doctor that maybe one of the reasons I kept passing out—and I don't mean swooning like a woman in an old black-and-white movie, I mean dropping like a sack of rocks—was because of a salt/water imbalance. Since the bird had just consumed a lot of salty crackers and I thought he might be thirsty, I walked over to a puddle of water in the middle of the parking lot, and he hopped along behind me. He dipped his beak into the rainwater and drank. I sprinkled some more crackers on the asphalt and he ate those, too, and then he drank some more, and then it was just me and the bird and the descending curtain of night and I thought, "Now what?"

The truth was that this bird was in a much more desperate state than I had realized two nights earlier. I knew he might die. I remembered that look on the small, scared faces of the birds my mother and I rescued. And so I let him decide what was best for him.

I cupped my hands together, forming a small nest, and rested them on the asphalt in front of the helpless creature. He cocked his head a little bit to the side, the way birds do when they are quizzical, and then, without any further hesitation, he hopped into my hands. Wild animals don't usually leap into our personal space, but this is exactly what happened, and in the weirdness of those pandemic times, it didn't really seem that unusual at all.

I stood up and held him inside my jacket, close to the warmth of my body. I hurried him home and made a soft place in a cardboard box the way my mother and I had all those times when I was a kid. I put a teacup full of water and a Club Cracker beside him, and I went to bed. For the first time since the pandemic began, I was not alone in my house.

FROM THE MOMENT Two-Step moved in, he was intent on going everywhere with me. As the maple leaves unfurled at the end of May 2020, we strolled along the sidewalk, Two-Step hopping beside me as we went around the block. There are a lot of stories I want to tell you about Two-Step: "Man Teaches Bird to Fly," "Pigeon Gets Struck by Car," "Bird Asks for Help in Bath." But it's late. I can't hold much more of this story in my head right now, so I need to stop talking to myself for now.

The pigeons and the dove are getting quiet. High up in the aerie the babies—it may just be one—are making some peeps. Two-Step is preening his primary feathers. I can hear the rhythmic soft sound as he pulls each one through his beak. These are the feathers that help him fly, and he is cleaning them and putting them in place. *Flik. Flik. Flik.* The sound is as steady as a heartbeat, and I set my breathing to it.

IN SOME WAYS I am fortunate. Since I was eight years old I have been telling myself stories this way. My childhood nighttime stories were so elaborate that I started going to bed earlier and earlier so I could revel in them (and reach a near-end) before falling asleep. Those stories were always about me performing some kind of heroic feat, sometimes surviving an airplane crash or making a great play on the baseball diamond, but mostly saving a girl—from a burning bus or a burning house or a burning forest. Something was almost always burning. Occasionally, there were floods, or blizzards, or terrorists (or all of the above). I suspect that the storytelling I did back then is why I am able to remember what I tell myself now, why I am able to hold these sentences in my head all night until I wake up and dictate them to my computer the following morning.

———

AFTER THE BIRD REHABILITATOR taught me how to rehabilitate Two-Step on my own, she gave me some tips on how to soft-release him. Of course, that depended on whether Two-Step got better, which she very much doubted. It may have been because I was so isolated—by circumstance and by illness—but getting Two-Step back into the wild, where he could experience the world the way a bird is supposed to experience the world, soon became pretty much all that mattered to me.

———

I POSTED SOMETHING about Two-Step on Facebook a few days ago. The occasion was January 5, National Bird Day. My hope was that the first post I had made in years—and my very first attempt at dictation—would be read by a few people, and they would donate to the bird charities I mentioned. It was intended to be a one-time thing, because I am a private person who pretty much never uses social media, but I still feel like I have more to say. In this pandemic, I think we are all feeling the preciousness of the world. I certainly am, but that may be because I am not sure how much longer I will be around.

Because of National Bird Day, I wanted to acknowledge how these creatures affect our lives. Sometimes just the sight of a bird or a flock of birds can lift you when you need it most—a mountain chickadee swooping toward the feeder, a black skimmer gliding low over the ocean, a cloud of starlings sweeping across a wintry blue sky. Sometimes a bird can be a hero, like Cher Ami, a messenger pigeon who in a single act of courage in World War I saved the lives of nearly two hundred American soldiers.

As I said in my Facebook post, there is a simple way to take care of the birds: keep your cats in the house and keep your plastics out of the ocean.

———

AFTER I BROUGHT Two-Step home, I was supposed to keep him in a box for about a week so that he wouldn't further injure himself, but thinking about him alone in the dark was just too heartbreaking, and I caved after two days. When I opened his box, he fluttered out, desperately seeking a safe place to land. He chose my head, not out of love, sadly, but because it was the highest (and thus safest) perch in the room.

Two-Step also enjoys perching on my outstretched arm when we go for a drive (yes, he loves riding in the car), which gives him a good view out the back window. He is fascinated by this perspective. Usually all I can see in the rearview mirror is his gorgeous butt and tail feathers, but sometimes he turns around and looks at the road in front of us, and when I see his face in the reflection, I am convinced he is bathing in the thrill of existence.

———

AS I LIE IN BED, telling myself this story, I wonder about Two-Step's life before he met me. I imagine he was born on or around the flat-roofed buildings that recently sprang up in the Sawmill District, which is named after the sawmills that used to line the adjacent Clark Fork River, which is named after William Clark, one half of the famous exploring duo (Lewis and Clark), the other half of which was Meriwether Lewis, the renowned naturalist who is responsible for one of only nine (nine!) official passenger-pigeon sightings in Montana, a big deal since the passenger pigeon didn't make it this far west very often, which must have happened before 1809, when Lewis killed himself in a Nashville inn, purportedly because he couldn't find a woman to spend his life with.

It is worth noting here that America was full of passenger pigeons at that time, all of them cousins of Two-Step. When I say "full," I mean that there were *three billion* passenger pigeons in this country, their flocks sometimes so big they would blot out the sky, but by September of 1914, when World War I was beginning, every single one of them was dead, hunted to oblivion. The very last passenger pigeon, Martha, died alone, of old age, isolated in her enclosure at the Cincinnati Zoo. Unlike so many of us, she had no choice but to die alone.

Cher Ami saved those American soldiers by carrying important military messages across enemy lines in a tube tied to his leg. After twelve successful missions, he got shot to shit and his right leg had to be amputated, ending his career. Cher Ami (whose name means "dear friend," a clever pun for a letter carrier, though maybe he and the other six hundred carrier pigeons flying above battlefields full of pissed-off German riflemen were not really so dear) died alone in captivity, too, though he is now not only an inductee in the Racing Pigeon Hall of Fame (yes, there is a hall of fame for pigeons), but people of all ages can visit the Smithsonian and gawk at his stuffed body.

I do need to apologize here to all the naturalists and historians and vast throngs of people who are much smarter than I am, because in recounting this, I am relying on the trivia I passively absorbed online a couple of years ago and which I can't revisit because looking at a computer screen with a migraine is itself an unthinkable act of bravery (and I'm no hero).

When I imagine the newborn that was Two-Step, I picture him in a nest on an east-facing balcony with some southern exposure (pigeons prefer to make nests that face south). Since pigeon clutches are almost always two eggs, Two-Step probably had an older sibling. With pigeons, the older sibling is the first to get food when the parents return to the nest and thus is bigger. Two-Step was small, still is, and I think if he were a bigger bird, he could have forced his way back into the nest and not been left to wander the mean streets (of Missoula, Montana!) waiting for me to come along.

———

WITH TWO-STEP SHARING MY HOME, I had to make a few adjustments. I converted my office (which was of no use to me anymore) into a sanctuary for him. I removed my literature textbooks and years of student grade books from the top of the bookcase and added ledges, using bricks and boards and large river rocks. I propped a four-foot mirror along the length of the highest roost (so that he could sit and admire the attractiveness of that other creature who looked just like him). I leaned another large mirror against the wall. (When I brushed my teeth, Two-Step would fly awkwardly up to my shoulder and we'd look in the bathroom mirror at ourselves. My hair hadn't been cut in months, my face was unshaven, and I had a wild bird on my shoulder, and as I looked at the two of us, I couldn't help but think that we were both broken.) I scattered objects across the floor, things I thought might interest a pigeon—a golf ball, a set of keys, some shower curtain rings, a bracelet that belonged to L., and a Beanie Baby bird that I picked up from a thrift store for two bucks that was about the same size as Two-Step. I took a drawer from an old bureau and put it in a large black trash bag, then went out to the yard and dug up a few square feet of sod, which I put in the drawer and set on the floor.

I watered the grass so it would grow lush and green and tall. My thinking was that Two-Step might want to occasionally hop in and walk around and feel the earth beneath his feet (foot).

Also, I covered everything—every surface in sight—with old sheets.

In those early days, I would occasionally tiptoe to my office doorway to check on Two-Step. He was usually contentedly looking at himself in the mirror. Sometimes he would be standing on his good leg, using his beak to pull at the curled, crippled toes on his bad foot, one at a time, trying to stretch them out.

This behavior baffled the bird rehabilitator; she said it wasn't something she had seen before, and she didn't expect it would help him get better. I knew that if he didn't get better, I couldn't return him to the wild. If he didn't get better, I would get to keep him.

But Two-Step kept tugging on his toes, and his leg started to straighten, though he still couldn't put weight on it. One morning when I got up and checked on him, he looked different. He was standing on one leg, but his toes were not curled up as tightly. They looked stronger and not just spindly and useless.

And a few days later, like the leaves on my boxelder maple tree in springtime, his toes began unfurling.

And a few days after that, his toes straightened out enough to allow him to plant his bad leg on a flat surface.

And then he began to walk.

I NAMED HIM TWO-STEP in part because when I first brought him home and he hopped around the yard, he took two steps with his good leg where other two-legged birds would take one. But his name also comes from a place on the Big Island of Hawaii, a snorkeling cove called Honaunau Bay that locals refer to as "Two Step," which L. and I visited many, many times.

As with rock climbing, where what is more important than figuring out how to get up is how to get down, with snorkeling sites like Two Step you need to figure out how you will get out of the water before you decide to go in. Just because you can get into the water without touching the corals or cutting up your hands or getting poisoned by an almost-too-pretty-to-look-at sea creature doesn't mean you will be able to get out. At Two Step, there is a spot where the lava rocks form two "steps" that make it possible to get in and out of the water, where you can see gorgeous walls of living coral and a spectacular array of tropical fish. Nearby, there are tide pools filled with miniature versions of the fish in the bay—tiny Moorish idols, tiny damselfish, maybe a tiny moray eel—and I spent hours gazing into them. Sometimes I'd be gazing into a tide pool at those fish and the reflection of the woman I loved would appear beside my own on the water's clear, still surface.

But for the first few months, I *never* used his name. Instead, I simply called him "Pigeon." When I went to his room to check on him, I'd say, "You okay, Pigeon?" Or when I imagined L. holding Two-Step in the palm of her hand for the first time, I'd imagine telling her, "I think Pigeon likes you."

In many cultures, parents wait because of fear or superstition to name a newborn child. I followed this practice, too, but I told myself it was because I didn't want to ever forget he was a bird of the wild—and not a pet. When people asked me his name, I said, "His name is Two-Step, but I call him Pigeon."

The truth is that I, like so many parents of newborn children, *was* terribly afraid that Two-Step was going to die, and I didn't think I could bear it. But something changed. One day, maybe six months in, I just couldn't call him "Pigeon" anymore, and he has been Two-Step ever since.

———

TWO-STEP WAS IMPROVING, but I wasn't. I noticed that my fists, especially while I slept, were getting more and more balled up. I always woke up stiff and sore all over, but the clenched fists were a troubling new symptom. Sometimes I'd imitate Two-Step pulling at his toes, holding out an arm, opening my hand, and pulling my fingers back as far as possible. It didn't seem to help.

I also suspected that I was experiencing seizures at nighttime. I couldn't know for sure, because they only happened when I was asleep, but on those mornings when I would wake up feeling particularly unrested and sore, I sensed it was because I'd had a seizure. I'd had them before. Years ago, my neurologist described them as "non-epileptic" seizures, likely harmless, but I now think they were pointing to whatever in my body was coming apart even then.

When I first experienced the seizures in the summer of 2011, the woman I loved was lying beside me. She would gently wake me with her soft, worried voice. "You're having one," she would say. And I'd whisper, "Thanks" and "It's okay." Oddly, I felt most rested, most at comfort, in the immediate aftermath of those nocturnal medical-mystery events. Partly, I know, because I got to revel in being cared for, watched over, protected. But since then, and especially during that first year of the pandemic, when so many of us were entirely isolated, I've wondered how people know if they are having a seizure. I've been told there is an app for this. You put your phone on the bed, and instead of your partner waking you up with a gentle touch and soothing words, your loveless device vibrates. It is your phone's language for telling you that you are alone, that you are sick, that something inside of you, deep down where the x-ray can't reach, is breaking.

THOUGH TWO-STEP WAS GETTING HEALTHIER and stronger, he showed little interest in flying. "You're a bird," I kept telling him. He didn't listen.

In the mornings, with my headache still blasting away, we would head outside for some fresh air. You'd think a bird given that kind of opportunity would take flight and soar to the heavens, but Two-Step just trailed behind me as I filled up the bird feeders and cleaned out the birdbaths and surveilled for evidence of the most murderous creatures to ever walk the planet earth: the neighbors' cats. Then I'd walk through the gate that led to the street and look back at Two-Step, and he'd seem kind of perplexed, like, "What's the big idea, where are you going?" But eventually he'd follow along and we'd take a leisurely stroll around the block.

Birds experience the world through their beaks, and Two-Step used his to pick up and sample every little thing he could find. We'd walk, then stop, walk, then stop, all around the block. If he became aware I was too far ahead of him, he'd scamper to catch up, but mostly we walked side by side, like an old married couple moving perfectly in step after supper on a warm summer evening. But my walks with Two-Step were also scary as hell. He was so small. Smaller than the dogs on the sidewalk, much smaller than the cars speeding by. He was even smaller than the squirrels. Standing next to the tall curb with a pebble in his mouth, he looked tiny, but the worst part was that he didn't seem aware of it.

This is why one of the first lessons I wanted to impart was making sure that Two-Step became afraid of cars. When the occasional car came by, I'd wait until it got close, then I'd clap my hands and do a wobbly "sprint" into a neighbor's yard. Sometimes Two-Step, alarmed, would take flight and follow me and land on my head, but most of the time he would just keep walking along the sidewalk without, as my mother used to say, a care in the

Buckbee & Fitzgerald

world. Because he had watched me fearlessly watering the grass out by the street while cars went by, he knew *I* was not scared of them. Pigeons are smart, and he had learned by studying me.

Another trick I used to get Two-Step flying was to coax him onto my head. I'd tap my head, and when he flew up I'd reward him with a peanut. If you were a neighbor of mine, I'm sure the gesture of me tapping my head furiously would have amused you. You might have said to your pandemic partner, "Is he trying to get a baseball player to steal second?" And your partner might laugh and say, "I think he's guiding a 747 to the Jetway." I, of course, would have been oblivious to both of you. I'd be drumming my aching head while still in my pajamas with my bird-dropping-stained baseball cap covering my many months of uncut hair, some toothpaste on this or that corner of my beard.

The real problem was that I, in a perversion of evolutionary justice, didn't know how to fly. Sure, I'd tried many times as a kid, but my flying was limited to making cardboard wings and jumping off the garage roof. What good was I to Two-Step? There were lots of nights when Two-Step would stand on my shoulder and we'd look into the mirror above the bathroom sink and I'd say, "I'm sorry I'm not a bird." Perhaps the bigger problem wasn't that I was not a bird but that he didn't realize he was one.

And so I started putting Two-Step in a milk crate and carrying him to the softball diamonds, and they were always deserted because even in a game of softball it is hard to maintain social distance by staying six feet away from everyone else. This was back when our very lives depended on staying away from everyone. Nevertheless, Parks & Rec watered the hell out of those fields that spring, pulling crisp mountain water right from the Clark Fork River (not more than a softball's throw away), which was rushing snowmelt toward the Idaho panhandle.

Two-Step enjoyed hop-walking around in the grass, even when it came up to his breastbone. "You dummy," I'd say affectionately to him. What I needed to do was make him *want* to fly. We'd be standing in left-center field—a place I used to call home when I was fleet-footed and sure of hand—and I'd clap and start sprinting toward center. Sometimes I'd look over my shoulder, and there would be Two-Step gracefully, effortlessly, flapping his wings and catching up to me, and thank goodness he was, because I'd quickly and completely run out of breath, slow down, hunch over, gulp for air, and he'd land on my head. He felt heavy as a bowling ball, the grip of his toes like screws in my scalp. But a few moments would pass, the black monster would subside a little, and I would catch my breath and attempt to dash toward right field, and Two-Step would fly after me. (Yes, in case you were wondering, I did flap my own arms while sprinting across the outfield grass.)

One summer night in the late 1990s, shortly after I arrived in Montana for grad school with a cheerful woman named Laurie (who I deeply loved, but not in the same way I loved L.), we went to the now-ghostly Go West Drive-In movie theater on Mullan Road to see the movie *Contact*. We sat on the hood of Laurie's car beneath a billion stars and watched a famous actress sit on the hood of her car beneath a billion stars. There's a line in the movie that has stuck with me, and it's what the scientist says when she is flying through outer space and trying to find the words to describe it: "They should have sent a poet."

I feel that way when I try to describe what it was like to watch Two-Step when he took flight. His first efforts were cautious as he flew in narrow circles around the park. When he was ready to land, he would look around for me, then drop down low and glide straight toward my head, pulling up at the last second with a furious flap of the wings before planting his two now-healthy taloned feet squarely on my baseball cap. (His aim in this regard would prove to be always perfect.) I'd hold some peanuts in my palm and he would walk down my arm and peck them up while standing in my hand, his throat pulsating from excitement, exhaustion, or both. He seemed to be vibrating, suddenly attuned to something that was completely invisible to me. I felt I was holding electricity, not dangerous but capable of bursting into blinding radiance at any moment. In a mere forty seconds, Two-Step had learned more about physics and aerodynamics than I could have if I studied it for the rest of my life.

And after days and days of rehearsal, he finally took off for real, and as his flight path widened, he flew higher and farther, scaring the living piss out of me when he disappeared from view. Eventually, though, I would see a dot in the sky, and then the dot would get bigger, fast. A pigeon can fly ninety miles an hour, and it can fly five hundred miles without a break, and if you drop one off at a location they have never been to before that is a thousand miles away, it may make its way back home before you do. But that is just science. What really happened is that a creature I had come to know (and I so loved him!) was flying for the first time, and it looked like it filled him with real, pure, true joy.

Sometimes when he got directly overhead and was flying against the wind, I'd see him in relief against the backdrop of a blue Montana summer sky, and he would seem to be completely still, not standing still but "flying still." And in those moments, all I wanted was for this bird to get a chance to do it all. Put his beak in a puff of snow in winter; feel the energy of the world as it comes alive in spring; meet a girl, fall in bird-love, and be with her forever.

———

MY DREAM FOR TWO-STEP now seemed possible. But though his health had rebounded, he still wasn't welcomed by the other birds. When he flew, he flew alone. And on those occasions when he would land on one of the cement beams of the bridge underpass, the other pigeons would chase him away or ignore him altogether (and it broke my heart). I would stand on the path below and hold out my hand, and when he was ready, he would come and land in my palm. His talons would grip my wrist or fingers and I'd let him rest there for as long as he wanted, no matter how bad my headache pulsed, no matter how fast the headache monster was closing in, no matter how badly my stomach twisted itself in knots when I needed to retch.

Then Two-Step would try again to be a bird, flying back up into the rafters, but again he would get bullied or left all alone. When he'd had enough, he would settle on my head, and I'd say to him, "Are you ready to go?" and if he didn't move for five or ten minutes, I'd say, "Let's go home."

———

I HAVE BEEN AFRAID to say it for months—even late at night in the dark of my bedroom.

It terrifies me really, but here it is:

I am a sick person.

Lately, the migraine has become the lesser of my problems, because now what is sometimes even worse is the symptom I have that is called "post-exertional malaise" (PEM). Not only do I have to endure the pain that comes with PEM, but my physical capacity is dwindling rapidly. My illness probably won't kill me, but people like me don't get better. I won't be cured and I won't improve. It will get worse until it can't get any worse, and I will live in that condition until I die.

I hate saying all this because, to me, there is nothing more pitiful than self-pity.

But my therapist (a word that used to be almost as bad to me as "self-pity") tells me I need to start coming out as a sick person.

She wants me to feel more comfortable with myself so that I will expand my connections and enjoy a more rewarding social life.

The truth is that the pandemic has been perfect camouflage. Everyone has been stuck in their homes, everyone has put their lives on hold, everyone is in pain. I've been able to hide from all of you.

So, yes, I am a sick person. I will not live the life I imagined. I won't do the things or see the places I've loved for so long. I won't play ice hockey again or swim out to the reefs. I won't hike that particular Rattlesnake Trail where I took the woman I loved, and where there is a giant ponderosa pine that's so beautiful I hugged it the last time I saw it. That tree—which I call the L. tree—will go unhugged, by me at least, forever. There's perhaps my favorite place in the whole wide world, not so far from town, that I also won't see again: a once-secret place in the Rattlesnake Wilderness, where the deep pools of cascading river water are baby blue, cold as steel, and the trout are longer than a pigeon's wingspan. And I will never walk into a classroom again and summon the force it takes to hold the attention of twenty-five minds for seventy-five minutes, willing them to think with power and joy for as long as they live.

I SUPPOSE IT doesn't really matter since we're in a pandemic, and everything is off-kilter (as my mother used to say), but I wear some pretty funny glasses these days. They are called FL-41S, and they clip on to my regular glasses and make me look like an inventor in an old sci-fi movie. They are tinted to help people with extreme light sensitivity, or photophobia.

The glasses supposedly block blue light waves, like those from fluorescent lights (which induce migraine). That's where the "FL" in the name comes from—"fluorescent." The "41"? I still have no idea. Are there FL-42 glasses that are even better? More likely, the number 41 was a random number made up by an ad department guy to make the glasses sound like a fancy car.

The vanity in me does not like them. At first, I wore them only on particularly bright days. You might think that means summer, but what it really means is winter. Snow is the enemy of the migraine sufferer. Fresh snow on a sunny day is the dinner bell of the black monster. You're like a pigeon surrounded by lip-smacking foxes—light up above, light down below, light in front of you (reflecting from the fallen snow that has collected on tree branches, mailboxes, car hoods, and the summer furniture you never got around to putting in the shed). Eventually, I had to start wearing the FL-41s every day, and now I wear them at night, which means my entire world is getting darker.

———

WE WERE SIX MONTHS into the pandemic, and people were acting goofy, erratic, dazed. The parking lot along the river was filled with cars that never moved, some with license plates from faraway places. I saw the same people every day. The same people walked their dogs and kept six feet apart; the same people jogged the same path, at the same pace, at the same time. Something dreamlike was happening to all of us.

Sometimes in the mornings on that trail by the flowing river with my bird on my aching head, it felt like there was no clear border between the dream world and the real world. It reminded me of the last long swim I took in an open body of water before I really got sick. It was a couple of years after things ended with L., and I had gone to visit my brother and his family in Chicago, and late one July night, I headed to Lake Michigan. (I went to the same beach I used to go to in high school, on Friday nights, with a girl I secretly loved—who I had saved from many a burning bus.) I had never seen the lake so still. It was like glass—or rather water in a glass, a glass that was on an end table in a dark family room while upstairs a mother and a father and a child slept, hugging their pillows, their windows open and curtains billowing in the shore breeze, the thunder of a storm in the distance, while downstairs a dreaming dog lay on his side on a cool tiled floor and kicked his legs, the tags of his collar brushing against the tile with a clinking sound that tiptoed through the quiet house, maybe looking for a dream to slip into, maybe shaking just slightly the leg of the table on which the glass of water rested, causing the surface of the water in the glass to roll, like a slow, steady breath that I slipped into.

The water was crystal cold, and though I was miles away from downtown Chicago, the combination of city light and starlight gave me a clear view of the sandy bottom in the shallows of the Great Lake. At first, I swam freestyle, an invisible woman by my side, trying to shake off the cold, and then, like a motorboat cutting its engine, I coasted and shifted to a breaststroke, one I could perform while barely disturbing the water. Straight out I swam, toward the enormous thunderheads that had gathered offshore, with the pink lightning making crooked paths through the towering clouds. When I dipped my head during my stroke I couldn't tell if my mouth was above the water or below—there was no gap in temperature between water and air—and I didn't know when it was safe to take a breath, I didn't know what was air and what was water, what was real and what was dream, if I was man or fish, or something in between.

———

I HAVE MORE DICTATED TEXT to polish, but I just can't look at the screen anymore. One of the absurdities of my illness is that when I look at lights too long my legs start to hurt.

I wanted to tell you about the three kinds of people that passed me under the bridge based on what they would say when they saw a pigeon on my head, but it will have to wait.

———

EVERY DAY, during my attempts to release Two-Step, I stood or crouched, Gollum-like, under the underpass of the Orange Street Bridge. Even in the shadows I was always wearing my clunky FL-41 clip-on glasses, my baseball cap pulled down low, my heavier-than-one-would-expect clothes, my bird flying from the rafters down to my head and back up again. We were a solid six months into our collective pandemic freak-out and even in the late morning—when my headache had receded a bit—there were a lot of joggers and bicyclists and walkers on this dirt offshoot of the Kim Williams Trail. The path was about eight feet wide, and on the river side were giant boulders to keep people and their little doggies from sliding down the riverbank into the Clark Fork River.

The joggers and bicyclists and walkers usually had one of three responses when they saw me and Two-Step. The joggers and bicyclists, without breaking pace, would often just say "cool." Others, the walkers usually, would look at us and stop, careful to keep a six-foot distance, and say, "Thanks, I needed that." These two responses happened over and over again. But there was also a third, equally frequent reaction. It almost always came from men, a certain kind of man that exuded a certain kind of disagreeable masculinity, and those men would roll their eyes and sneer at us while making a sound like *pfft*.

I could recognize myself in all three of these kinds of passersby, and the one that stood out, because it made me feel ashamed, was the last. I think these men enjoyed seeing me with a bird on my head and contraption-glasses on my face because it made them feel better about themselves. I can imagine those men were thinking, "What a loser. He could be out riding a bike, or jogging or swimming, or drinking a bunch of beers with friends, but instead he's looking for attention by standing under a bridge with a bird on his head."

They didn't know, of course, that I couldn't be out jogging or biking and I couldn't hang out with my friends. I wanted to tell these men, "I used to ride my bike from my front porch step into the Rattlesnake, deeper into the wilderness than you've ever gone." I wanted to point at the river and yell, "I used to swim in that river." And when I say "swim," what I mean is that I would wade in with my goggles, find a current that was the right pace, and swim against it for hours without moving an inch. I was like a fish in water (or a pigeon in the sky).

But now I couldn't even swim across a pool without getting extreme post-exertional malaise. The fish in me was dead, the hockey player was dead, the teacher was dead, the romantic partner was dead. I was now a guy sitting on his couch in his pajamas and an old hat, everything around him covered with stained thrift-store sheets.

Some of the strangers on the path did stop to ask questions, and I told them about Two-Step and all the pigeon life under that bridge, pigeons they probably walked right past without seeing (or worse, looked at with disgust). Maybe they had some prejudice against pigeons, but I believe that was gone after talking to me. I had become an ambassador of what someone in a movie cruelly called "a rat with wings." I didn't talk about my own health issues, though I would have a migraine and my stomach would be roiling, and when Two-Step would land on my head, I would calculate how many hours and minutes before the sun-demon sank beneath the horizon and I could get into bed and turn out the lights.

The people who stopped to talk provided me with a much-needed feeling of connection. And they didn't deter Two-Step whatsoever. I could be standing there talking to a group of people for fifteen minutes and Two-Step might not leave my head even once. Sometimes I'd teach small children how to hold out their hands so that Two-Step would fly onto their little arms and gently peck up some peanut pieces from their palms. "It's okay," I'd tell the little kids (and their moms and dads). "He won't hurt you." And during that strange time those strangers would trust this strange man because, well, why the hell not, considering.

My headache was relentless and the doctors I went to would usually ask if I was seeing a psychiatrist yet. They were accustomed to seeing symptoms they understood and people they could fix, and I wasn't one of those. I was desperate to escape the pain. One evening, when I was coming close to the end of my rope, I decided to go to the Buddhist center one block from my house. It was there I learned the concept of the two darts.

From what I gathered, the Buddha described getting hit by a dart and feeling great physical pain. But then he talked about the second dart, which was even worse. The second dart is the thinking we do in response to our pain. "Will I get hit by more darts? Was it a mistake to go for a walk alone? What if I get gangrene and I have to get this thing sawed off? Why don't people like me? When is this suffering going to end?" And so on.

I bring this up now only to draw attention to the obvious. And as a way to honor all those kind people who stopped to talk to a stranger about the bird on his head. It was a time of loneliness, an epidemic of loneliness. Disease isolates. Pain isolates. And when you need comfort the most, that is when it's hardest to find. But then the strangers arrive, brought to you as a result of the cosmic intersection of pandemic and bird. And so I want to finish with something else I heard frequently. After stopping to chat, many people, both women and men (including, sometimes, that sneering type of masculine man), would say these three words: "It's a blessing." I would hear those words and nod, but it took me a while to fully understand what they really meant.

Buckbee & Fitzgerald

Part 2

WHEN YOU HAVE A MYSTERY ILLNESS, WELL-INTENTIONED people will try to help you with diagnoses of their own. So I need to tell you, before you offer suggestions, that I have been tested for everything the doctors can think of. I've been poked and prodded and scanned, and my blood and spinal fluid and urine have been analyzed, and I've gotten MRIs and X-rays and CT scans. I have been weighed over and over, like a suspicious-looking truck crossing a border. I have taken this pill and that pill and gotten this shot and that shot. I've had needles stuck in my arms and head and face. I have been injected with toxins. There seems to be consensus about what I don't have. I don't have Lyme disease. I don't have bird flu. I don't have Ehlers-Danlos or Sjögren's. I don't have Guillain-Barré, and I don't have ankylosing spondylitis. I don't have a brain lesion. And my cerebrospinal fluid isn't leaking in the slightest.

People advise me to sleep more. But if I don't get out of bed when my headache wakes me up, it will certainly turn into a migraine. (And my migraines, like clockwork, for whatever reason, always last thirty-six hours.) Just feeling the kind of tiredness you can't shake off no matter what you do will trigger a migraine. And naps are simply not an option, because any nap, whether five minutes or two hours, is almost certain to trigger a migraine.

I would like to list the drugs I have taken, but I don't remember all of them. I would like to consult my eight-hundred-page medical history, but I can barely pick it up, much less pore over it. The standout memory of a multiday visit to multiple buildings at the Mayo Clinic campus in Minnesota is the melodious word everyone kept repeating like a mantra: *gabapentin, gabapentin, gabapentin*. Traveling is not easy when you're in pain, but I made the 1,200-mile journey to that renowned medical center only to have the specialists recommend a medication I'd already tried that didn't work. And I am not alone in all this confusion.

The Mayo Clinic concluded I have something called central sensitization, which is basically what other people call chronic fatigue syndrome. But because chronic fatigue syndrome basically sounds like you are tired, advocates prefer to use the term "myalgic encephalomyelitis" (the acronym is ME/CFS). According to the Centers for Disease Control, anywhere from 836,000 to 2.5 million Americans have ME/CFS. I don't know why that range is so vast. At least one-quarter of those individuals are bedbound or housebound and will never regain their previous level of functioning. It hurts to think about all those people who are suffering, and it also hurts to think about all the silence (and misinformation) around them. I have spent years researching ME/CFS, feeling briefly hopeful about this or that promising study or protocol, but there is still no cure. There is not even a diagnostic test.

I NEED TO TAKE you back to the year 1974. Watergate was about to rub out Nixon, Larry Bird was breaking his French Lick high school's all-time scoring record, the movie *The Exorcist* was number one at the box office, and a ratty-looking, audacious twenty-four-year-old musician told his friends he was going to make the best rock 'n' roll album ever. One line in the first track of the album he made has been rolling around in my head lately. When I'm dictating or polishing what I dictated, I hear it; when I crawl under the covers at night and tell myself the next part of the story, I hear it; when I sit in the stillness of my room listening to the soft clicking noise of the birds' toes on the kitchen linoleum floor, I hear it. I can't stop hearing it. The line is: "Well now, I'm no hero, that's understood."

One of the rules in fiction writing is to beat the absolute living hell out of your main character. Have him lose his car keys, get shingles, be afraid of the water. A lightning strike is a good idea. Even better, make the character's own flaws beat him up. As a result of his own rage, he loses his job. As a result of his own weakness, the girl he loves leaves him. Two-Step, for instance, got abandoned, broke his leg, got hit by a car, and was ostracized by his own peers. He's easy to root for. (Plus, he is so handsome. He is the hero of this story.)

But this isn't fiction, and I'm not trying to get you to root for me, and I'm not trying to manufacture some kind of narrative tension. I just want to get this story out while I still can.

The musician I was speaking of was Bruce Springsteen, and the album was *Born to Run*, and the song was "Thunder Road."

I once knew a boy who fell in love with Bruce Springsteen. The boy was at an age when you wouldn't think he would be interested in a song like "Thunder Road," but he loved dancing wildly to it. I joined in and danced along with him, and when the song ended, we would play it again. We danced together as the song played over and over until it was time for dinner. And no matter how long I danced with him, I never got weak or out of breath, and I never got a headache or post-exertional malaise. That stuff would come later.

There is optimism and hope in the album *Born to Run*, but there is also an increasing sense of darkness. Springsteen's music was changing in a way that would be especially evident a couple of years later when he released his next album, the aptly titled *Darkness on the Edge of Town*. As an adult, Springsteen has suffered from depression, and it drips off that album and all that followed, even the fuel-injected *Born in the USA*. And, well, I'm no music critic, that's understood, but I have had loss—a father who died way too young; a mother who died way too young; loves lost; friends lost; and the list goes on, as I'm sure it does for you, too. And maybe I am trying to avoid talking about all of that, the darkness on the edge of things.

———

I'M HAPPY TO REPORT that Two-Step and V. are rather busy these days. They have two new babies. Three weeks ago, at hatching time, the baby pigeons were each the size of my thumb, with gigantic closed eyes and soft yellow wisps of fuzz. Now they are as big as baseballs, their eyes are open and focused, and the yellow fuzz has been replaced with pinfeathers (undeveloped feathers that make them look like porcupines). In a week or so, the pinfeathers will fill out and look like real feathers, and then each baby will be big enough to be confused with a small adult. You would not believe how fast pigeons grow.

———

ONE MORNING LATE LAST SPRING, Two-Step's second spring with me, I woke up to a silent house with a shocking amount of light coming through my (supposedly) blackout shade. I immediately went into panic mode.

Normally, Two-Step woke me shortly after dawn by squawking from the other side of my closed bedroom door. Though Two-Step spent his days in the shed-hutch with his growing family, he always insisted on sleeping in the house. (And before long I brought them all in and let them stay in the house with me.) When I heard him, I'd get out of bed, go into the living room, and watch the blessing that was my pandemic buddy fly from one perch to the next, always in the same order, until finally alighting atop the refrigerator, which is right next to the front door. All I had to do was put on a cap and my contraption-glasses and crouch down beside the refrigerator, and then Two-Step would step right onto my head. We'd walk out into the yard and I'd give a quick scan for cats, then we'd head toward the shed and Two-Step would fly to the hutch, waddle through the little entrance, and disappear inside with his family. I'd go back in my now-empty house, take my meds, and sit on the couch and wait for my headache to recede enough so I could function.

But on this particular morning, I hadn't heard a peep from Two-Step. When I got out of bed and went into the living room, I found him on the shelf high up by the ceiling. He was standing on one leg, teetering a little. His feathers were puffed up, his head was pulled down into his body, and his eyelids were closed. I had never seen him like this, and it scared the hell out of me.

But I had overreacted before, like the night he didn't come home, or the time I couldn't find him in the house. Or that time he got hit by the car and was catapulted into the hedge that bordered the irrigation ditch. So I tried to hold it together. I stepped onto a stool and scooped him up—he didn't resist in the least—and I put him on the coffee table in front of me, where he assumed the exact same posture. I decided if he didn't show improvement in an hour, I would call the vet. I put some peanuts in front of him, but he didn't give them a look.

CxwszA

(Hey! Two-Step just walked across my laptop keyboard while I was dictating! That's what he wrote. That is Two-Step's first word! What is he trying to say to us? What is on his mind? What I find most impressive is how he somehow bracketed his word with uppercase letters. He's so smart.)

As the hour passed and Two-Step hadn't moved, I began to freak out. At eight thirty, I called the vet. I said, "My bird, Two-Step, is sick, can I bring him in?" I intentionally referred to him as my "bird," so that the vet assistants might assume I was speaking about a parrot or cockatoo—an "important" bird and not an "invasive species." (Plus, I had learned from TV hostage dramas that using a real name could elicit more sympathy.)

They told me the bird doc had surgeries scheduled all day, but if I could get there in twenty minutes, she would give him a look.

I don't know how I did it. Somehow, I suddenly had my keys and wallet and dashed out to the shed with Two-Step tucked in the crook of my arm. I found the pet carrier that had been used ten years earlier when I took my mom's cat Missy for her last car ride, and I laid a blanket on the bottom of the pet carrier, gently placed Two-Step inside, latched the door, speed-walked across the lawn to the car, got in, and did a tight U-turn on my street so I could get to the main road more quickly.

At first, the speed limit was twenty-five, and I went forty. Then the speed limit was thirty, and I went sixty. When it turned to sixty, I went ninety-five. That's when I spotted a police car on an intersecting street. I tried to decide what I would do when the cop came after me. I could pull over, point to the pet carrier, and say, "It's a life-or-death trip to the vet." And the cop would say, "What's in there?" And I'd lie like hell. "My doggie," I'd say.

More likely, though, I knew, I wouldn't stop at all. I'd speed all the way, with the cherry-top behind me, and turn into the vet's parking lot, kicking up gravel and dust. I'd assume the cops would know what I was doing, but maybe they wouldn't. Maybe when I stepped out of the car with the pet carrier in hand, they'd fire off a couple of rounds. Maybe I would collapse to the asphalt, dropping the pet carrier, and the latch would pop and Two-Step would fly out—completely healthy again, no longer in need of me—and soar toward the heavens alongside the spirit from my now-dead body.

MOST PEOPLE FEEL NEEDED. They have a partner and kids who depend on them, or they have a job that gives them meaning (and maybe helps others). Maybe they are part of a team or a club or a fan base. But what happens when they are no longer needed? Do they start to have a thought they've never had before: "Is there really a reason I need to be around?" One night last fall something happened that caused me to have that thought for the first time.

The brazen neighborhood cats had learned that once it got near dark, they could slip into my yard and, well, act like cats. I think they were trying to provoke me, like young neighborhood kids do to the old guy who lives in the house where the lawn has gone unmown, the leaves are never raked, and the shutters are falling off.

This is why I had gotten in the habit of tiptoeing out of my house in the near-dark to listen for slight disturbances in the brambly bushes that surround my yard. (Now I sound like a crazy person, yes?) If I heard a noise, I would run right at it even if I couldn't see the cat that was making the noise. My goal was to scare it to near-death so that it would have ingrained in its tiny, adorable skull that it needed to stay away from my birds. These short little sprints were also enough to jolt awake the headache monster and ignite a full-blown migraine, but if I wanted to protect the perimeter, I really had no choice.

One night, when I heard the familiar rustling of bushes and crunching of leaves, I dashed straight at the noise, and it was only when I got about twelve feet away and the animal backed out of the bushes and raised itself up that I realized it wasn't a cat at all. It was a bear, a black bear, a *big* black bear. There were silver reflections of light in his fur, and he possessed the formidable brawn that is particular to bears. I don't think I saw his claws, but I could see them clearly in my mind. As we eyeballed each other, the feeling I had was one of awe—he was so beautiful.

Every year in Montana it was my mission to lay eyes on at least one bear, and when it was summer and I was fly-fishing deep in the wilderness, or it was fall and I was hiking in the Rattlesnake, I'd get my fix, and though perhaps reckless, I tended to think the nearer to the bear the better. But now I couldn't hike, and I couldn't get into the wilderness, and the summer was over, and I hadn't seen a bear. Yet one had come to my house. Why had that bear come to visit me? Had I willed him into my yard? Was the universe sending me a message? I'd like to think it was something like that, but in reality the bear probably came into the yard because my yard was littered with birdseed. So I guess, in a roundabout way, that bear was a gift from Two-Step.

I was aware the bear was using that moment to make a choice—to either sprint right at me and separate my head from my body or to scamper up a tree. If I were needed by anyone—if I had a child or if I had the woman I loved—I wouldn't have felt calm; if I had students, I wouldn't have felt calm. I had Two-Step, of course, but he had his beloved V. And so I *did* feel calm. If the bear came at me, well, that wouldn't be such a bad way to go. I could imagine the high school reunion: "What happened to Buckbee?" "Oh, he got eaten by a bear."

But the bear did not run after me, and months later, when I raced to the vet, the cop did not chase me down. I rushed Two-Step into the clinic and they signed me in and, because of the pandemic, I waited outside. I placed the carrier on a bench and knelt down so I could talk to Two-Step and look at the intake person through the glass door at the same time. "You're going to be okay," I said over and over again. I don't know if this mantra soothed him at all, and I guess it was probably meant more for me anyway. I needed him to be okay. And why?

Because I loved my bird.

When we got called into the examination room, the vet gave Two-Step a quick look-over and asked me if I had any droppings from him. On the drive over, that small, helpless, sick creature had produced something so foul I had been forced to roll down the windows. But it was also fortunate, because it allowed the vet—Dr. Card is her name, and she is a very special human being—to gather a sample. She told me she needed to go to the lab and look at it under a microscope. Two-Step, the growing headache monster, and I waited in that tiny room. I was a sick person in a pandemic, still wearing the clothes I'd slept in, talking to a pigeon I was sure was going to die. I felt totally, utterly alone. How could Two-Step leave me? Didn't he know what that would do to me?

Two-Step and I waited in the small examination room for the vet to return, and I was struggling to hold it together. I'd had previous experiences in this same kind of small room where the doctor is about to anoint you with a crown of grief.

When I was twenty-one, a doctor looked me right in the eye and said, "Your father is going to die."

I was also in a small room like this when a doctor sitting across a desk from me said three impossible, unendurable words about my still-young mom, who I loved so much. "She has Alzheimer's."

Bad things happen in these small rooms. As I sat on the low, little stool by the exam table, I talked to Two-Step. "You're going to be home soon," I told him. "We're going home." Home, that's what mattered most, no matter what the doctor said.

We didn't have to wait long for Dr. Card to return. When she did, she had an answer. "He has salmonella."

And I tried not to break down in tears—me, a grown man with a pigeon—while the vet told me that Two-Step might be fine. She showed me how to use a syringe to plunge the antibiotic between Two-Step's wedged-open beak. She told me that— even if he was passing the salmonella to his babies when he fed them—this might actually be *good* for their immune systems, and now, if the babies were indeed sick, he would be passing on the antibiotic to them, as well. So much reason for hope. But I felt the fragility of the whole world, the awareness of how things you thought you could count on could be destroyed in a second.

I had two questions for the vet I knew I had to ask, but I was having a hard time speaking because I was on the precipice of bawling. The questions were the same questions I had been asking caregivers at the end of my visits for the previous two years, whether it was my rheumatologists or neurologists or massage therapists or osteopath or gastroenterologist or naturopath or my GP or the people from U of U Health in Salt Lake or the Mayo Clinic in Minneapolis.

Dr. Card, to her credit, was patient, though this was her surgery day. She probably had the lives of half a dozen birds depending on her. But she waited until I stopped gulping for air long enough to form a sentence without having a total meltdown: "What should I be on the lookout for over the next few days that would necessitate me reaching out to you?" She told me to check Two-Step's food bowl and his water bowl to make sure he was eating and drinking and also to let her know if he was still puffing out his plumage. The way she talked reminded me of my father's oncologist. She kind of looked at me sideways, as if she recognized she was dealing with an extreme case, somebody who was not responding to the situation like a normal person would. She was maybe thinking, "For whatever reason, to this man, this pigeon is more than just a pigeon." She reached for a sticky pad, wrote something down, handed it to me, and said, "Here, this is my home number."

The people in this world! You have met them. You have been them. God bless you and them.

The second question I had an even harder time voicing. The doctor waited through several false starts before I could get the words out: "Isn't there anything else I can do?"

But there was nothing else I could do.

By that point, on that day when I visited the vet, I had had the same headache for 792 days. As for the rest of my health, I felt like a cartoon character hanging on to the roots growing from the side of a crumbling cliff.

The reminder of impermanence was overwhelming. It brought back the other losses, all of them at once. My father who was overcome by cancer, my mother who I spoon-fed near the end, L. and the Springsteen-loving child who disappeared from my life, the bird who might not get to live his life. I would probably never get to see the tide pools again, or have a drink at a bar with a lovable woman, or skate with the puck through a pair of defenders.

I carried Two-Step out of the vet's office and put him in my car. I wanted to get him home as quickly as possible so he could be as comfortable as possible, but I had to pull over on the side of Highway 93 so the dam inside me could break open.

When I was able to compose myself, I started the car up again. I drove past landmarks that brought back memories—the motel where I'd spent the night with the woman I loved, the fairgrounds where I'd skated on the hockey rink, the school playground I'd visited with the boy who had disappeared.

Later, in the quiet of my house at dusk, I thought of all my friends who were suffering, all my friends who were having a hard time. I sat on my couch, took the heavy glasses off my aching face, and pulled my hand-knit beanie down over my eyes to block the dying light, surrounded by birds at peace preening their feathers and baby pigeons who poked their heads over the ledge, wondering what it would be like to step out into the enormous world.

———

TO GIVE TWO-STEP his antibiotic I had to swaddle him in a cloth and place him on a high table that in different circumstances could have served as a diaper-changing station. If I covered his eyes with the cloth, he wouldn't resist too much, but still I had to lean my chest on top of him to keep him in place while I pried open his beak and pressed the plunger of the syringe. I had to be careful to inject the medicine in the corner of his mouth—not the center, because that is where his air passage is, and if I got the medicine in the wrong part, I could drown him.

With each passing day it became more difficult to give Two-Step his medicine, and that was a good sign because it meant he was getting stronger, he was regaining his vitality, and he was returning to his old self. I routinely checked on the babies in the shed-hutch and they showed no signs of ill health, nor did V. Unlike all of them, however, I wasn't doing so good.

The pandemic rolled on, and we were in that exciting time of late spring, after the plum trees had blossomed so ferociously it looked like they were covered with freshly fallen snow and before the wild rosebushes—the same ones that hid the bear that could have killed me—would explode into yellow fireworks overnight. We'd had a lot of light rains, so the yard was plush with lushness. A large doe had been visiting, having smelled the birdseed from the zillion bird feeders I had put out, but she wasn't so large any-more. Now she had two sparkling new fawns with her, big-eyed, white-spotted, wet-nosed, heartbreaking in their vulnerability.

My bird craziness was not limited to the feeders. I had also visited the Lowe's website and seen plastic saucer sleds listed at an insanely low price. The website said my local store had eleven of them, but when I arrived at the store, the clerk told me they had put the sleds away until next winter. (I imagined her think-ing, "What idiot wants to buy sleds in May?" And me saying in response, "The idiot that is me.")

We toured the garden section, our necks craned back and to the side, the way Two-Step holds his head when his keen golden-irised eye scans the sky for hawks and falcons, until we found the sleds. They were wrapped in plastic, about two stories up on the uppermost shelf. The clerk looked at me as if I was asking the impossible, as if we were at the base of El Capitan.

But I wanted those sleds, so she found the guy who was licensed to operate the amazing machine that could reach those great heights. At one point, when the machine got stuck between two rows, I was sure the shelves would be knocked over and everything would tumble everywhere, but he managed to fork the pallet and bring the saucer sleds down. All the while, the sparrows and finches that had taken up residence inside the store were flittering around us.

"How many do you want?" the machine operator asked me.

"Just one," I said.

He looked like he was going to punch me. I guess with my surgical mask on he couldn't tell I was joking. The pandemic was death to those of us with a dry sense of humor. "I'll take seven," I said. And just like that, I had seven new birdbaths.

I set up several of them beneath my ancient boxelder maple tree, filling them with water and putting large river rocks in some of them and small river rocks in the others. I lay branches across the top. I'd later learn that what I was doing wasn't very hygienic for the birds (since it provided an inviting place for them to perch while relieving themselves), but the finches and sparrows and chickadees and nuthatches—and the pigeons, of course—loved those sleds.

At times, in my fenced-in yard, completely obscured from the street and neighbors by the bushes around the perimeter, I felt like I was living in a zoo enclosure. The coronavirus couldn't get to me, but neither could the UPS guy.

In the morning, when I sat on my one-step stoop, bent over, my aching head in my hands, sometimes I'd raise my head and find a baby deer sniffing near my toes, or I'd feel the tap of a chickadee as it landed on my shoulder.

Next to the stoop, partially under the branches of the box-elder, I had set up a six-foot folding ladder for Two-Step to use as a perch. He liked to stand on the top (warning: not a step!), where he could be close to the front door, see over a corner of the roof, keep an eye on the shed-hutch where his firstborns lived, and be protected from predators. I think he was also comfortable there because the top of the ladder was next to the branch he sat on at dusk while waiting for me to return from my class at the Buddhist center.

————

ONE OF THE REGULAR FEATURES of the beginners' Buddhism class was a sitting meditation, and whenever we got to that part, I would get up and go for a walk around the block. No way was I going to do a "body scan" or investigate my mind by using my breathing as an "anchor." I wanted to move away from—not toward—my body.

The fellow who runs the class—Sthiradasa—is a musician and scientist, a decade older than I am, an incredibly gifted listener, and though he has been ordained by his Buddhist sect, he doesn't consider himself a monk. He was just as astute as Two-Step's veterinarian, however, because he recognized I was in a not-so-good place and generously offered to meet with me weekly to see if he could find a way to help me get relief.

During those meetings, we didn't chant, wear robes, or burn incense. There were no gongs or bowls that sang. He asked about my challenges, and I learned about his, and he told me that Buddhism had a built-in flexibility I could take advantage of. One time, he advised me to stay open. "The relief may come in a way you don't expect," he said.

A few weeks after that conversation, I was in the yard with Two-Step. It had just started to drizzle. There were no cats in sight. Two-Step was flying from perch to perch—my roof, my neighbor's roof, the boxelder tree limb, etc. The fawns were hiding, one beneath the rosebushes, the other in my perennials beside the oversized thistle plant. For some reason I decided to climb the ladder. It wasn't easy in my condition.

I was fully aware that I was borrowing Two-Step's spot. I thought of all the times he sat there, or stood there, my bird, who was so slow to release to the wild. He liked to bathe in the light rain, lifting up first one wing to the sky and then the other. And now I was the one in the light rain, sitting on the DANGER step, my head amid the lower branches of the old tree. I don't want to say I became a bird, which sounds ridiculous, but it felt like I became birdlike. These were desperate times, pandemic times, and I had been instructed to be open to something new, and the image of myself that had been recurring in my mind for some time was of a spacecraft hurtling toward earth and shedding parts, one piece after the next, being stripped down to next to nothing along the way.

I closed my eyes and heard the sounds of my neighborhood, especially the birds that were visiting the feeders and baths, singing to one another as they ate and drank and bathed, but also the dog from a few doors down barking, and the overhead door of a distant delivery truck slamming shut, and the wind nudging the way-high-up leaves of the neighbor's narrowleaf cottonwood tree. I felt an expansive sensation and an awareness that my place in this landscape was small and that these same birds—even the "common" pigeons like Two-Step—had been doing this same thing in this same place for thousands of years, millions of years, before anything that looked like me walked here.

People under the pigeon bridge, where I had tried to soft-release Two-Step, had told me over and over again that he was a blessing. And now I understood the full extent of what they meant.

The birds were in my yard because of Two-Step, the deer because of Two-Step, Two-Step because of Two-Step, and I was on the ladder because of Two-Step. I realized that I was going to be able to hold on. And I don't mean anything dramatic, like my life was in the balance or anything like that, I just mean that I knew I would be able to hold on to my worldview, the same one I had as a child when my mother and I were saving the little birds, the same worldview I had when I roamed the streets of my hometown in junior high, knocking on the doors of the girls I liked, the same worldview I had when I swam alone on the glass surface of the Great Lake toward the massive electric clouds. Despite everything I'd lost, what was most important remained. You could hardly call the gifts Two-Step had given me common.

———

THIS MORNING, one of Two-Step's babies left the nest in the living room for the first time and flew to the shelf behind the couch. I tilted my head back and looked up and saw three pigeon heads peering down at me—Two-Step, V., and their baby.

Soon the weather will be warm, the days long. The lilac will start budding and the parade of spring will begin. The deer will shed their winter coats and the northern flicker will bathe in a puddle of melting snow. I am constructing a nesting box for Two-Step and V. that I will attach to the outside of my living room window. When it is warm enough, I will move their eggs into it, and Two-Step will leave the house to care for them. He probably won't want to come back inside the house. And then I will be able to watch him through my window, this not-so-common common rock pigeon, the bird the passersby called a blessing, my pandemic buddy, and alone in my room of echoes, I will know that he and I have completed the softest of releases.

WHEN THE DOCTOR at the hospital told me that my father was going to die, I was twenty-one years old. At that moment, my father was on an upper floor, getting chemo for the aggressive cancer that had suddenly invaded his mouth and brain, and I suppose on some level I knew the situation was dire.

But I didn't know if I *wanted* to know how dire. And I didn't know if there were certain emotions I should convey. Should tears be involved? Noisy remonstrations? I was overwhelmed with the self-consciousness that has afflicted me since childhood and did what came easiest. Not a tear, not a whimper. What the doctor got from me was a stone face. If my father had seen me, he probably would have been proud.

I was living in Chicago that spring, working three jobs (one for rent money, one for college money, and one for "beer" money). I had a double-shift job as a waiter at a private dining club in the Sears Tower. My graveyard shift was at the Hyatt Regency, the one that's famous for having the longest freestanding bar on the continent. In addition to those eighty hours a week, I sometimes worked as a vendor at Wrigley Field, selling peanuts and Pepsi. Making money was unusually important to me from an early age, partly because my father didn't have a steady—or at some points, any—income.

At the Hyatt Regency's twenty-four-hour restaurant, there seemed to be a nightly contest between the cooks and the guests to see who could drink more alcohol and inhale more cocaine. If you were a guest at 3:00 AM, you might wait two hours for a steak. Or you might get it in eight minutes. I had promised myself I would work forty shifts before quitting. That number always had a biblical resonance to me, and I figured that was about as long as my father had left to live.

Because I was young and healthy, I could survive on only a few hours of sleep each night. But I was tired, and my legs were heavy, and my eyelids were heavy, and my feet were killing me from walking on the restaurant's hard stone floors in used wing-tip shoes that were older than I was. I didn't have time to wash my uniforms, so I would usually toss them in the dryer to freshen them up with a dryer sheet. One morning, the manager pointed at me during our daily inspection and said, "What's that?" The other servers turned to look at me and laughed. I lifted up my arm and saw that one of my black dress socks was static-clung to the side of my white tuxedo shirt.

On the way to my three jobs, I slept on the train, sometimes by accident, sometimes on purpose. I worked in the famous Loop of Chicago, and so if I missed my stop, I could stay on the train and wait for it to go around its "loop."

After my graveyard shift, I would go to the edge of the Chicago River, sit on a wall, and put the orange-padded Walkman headphones over my ears. I listened to Sinéad O'Connor sing "Nothing Compares 2 U" again and again while looking down at the city lights shimmering off the choppy water. Some clever engineer a century earlier decided this river should start running in the opposite direction so that the water polluted by the local residents and factories would flow out of the state by way of the Mississippi River and eventually into the Gulf of Mexico, and not into Lake Michigan (where, twenty-five years later, I swam in those cleaned-up clear waters at midnight). The Chicago River now runs backwards, and as I sat there staring at it, I would think, "How many lives of ducks and birds and fish did that man ruin?"

The wall was about twenty feet above the river, and behind me was a slick glass-and-steel tower designed by the famous architect Mies van der Rohe: the IBM Building. To my right were the Marina City towers, where lots of TV shows and movies were filmed, including one with Steve McQueen (who, like

Buckbee & Fitzgerald

my father, would die from cancer at the age of fifty). The city was mostly quiet and sleepy until the newspaper-laden trucks would begin to pour forth from the underbelly of the *Sun-Times* building like ants from a disturbed anthill. I thought about my father. His disappointment in me as a young teen had recently started to change, and it seemed terribly unfair that just as we were becoming friends he was going to die.

It was a gorgeous early-spring day when my father was buried. The leaves on the trees were green. The flowers were bright. The sky was blue.

IT TOOK ABOUT A YEAR for my father to die, but when L. dropped out of my life, it took less than ten minutes. We had recently moved into our new home, proclaimed ourselves a family, our private wedding ceremony was imminent, and we were fresh off visits to friends and family—in Chicago, Colorado, and Texas—where we had pre-wedding receptions with the people we loved. L. came over as I was packing up the rest of my belongings at my old house. The sun was shining that spring day, too. The leaves were green. The flowers were bright. The sky was blue. She said she needed to talk about something real quick. And then she pulled a string that opened the curtain to a fateful world I didn't know existed.

In the ruins of our relationship, I quickly found a therapist and began seeing her three times a week (sometimes four). I kept telling her, "It feels like gravity has stopped working." Before each appointment, while I waited for the therapist's door to finally open, I would walk laps around and around the halls on the third floor of the building where she worked. That first summer without L. was a hot one, and in late July I began wearing my quick-dry shorts and water shoes to my appointments. When our time was up (always too soon), I would walk down the stairs and out to the street and then I'd walk two blocks to the edge of the Clark Fork River and, without breaking stride, I'd step into the river, pull my shirt over my head, stuff it in my shorts pocket, find the current, and start floating home.

If people were looking at the river from one of the downtown bridges, they might have seen me drifting past. Not in a boat or an inner tube but on my back and bum, a passenger "seated" in a river that flows in its God-given direction. They may have thought, "Oh, that looks like fun."

I couldn't exactly call the water that tumbled by the big river rocks "rapids," but the chop was rough enough to occasionally push my head beneath the surface or slap my face. It wasn't always a smooth ride, and I welcomed that.

There were usually some ducks in the river with me. I thought of them as "scooters." They were smaller and more slender than the mallards that congregated there, and they had the ability to walk, or "scoot," on top of the water for several yards at a time. I'm not sure why, but I liked to think it was a form of play.

Sometimes they'd join me in the current and we'd float together downstream. Then they would all suddenly dive beneath the surface, and I'd wait for them to pop up ahead of me like corks—first one, then the next, and so on, in rapid succession. When that happened, I would paddle quickly with my hands to try and catch up with them.

When I floated under the shadows of the bridges, I'd feel a blast of cool air and hear the water smacking against the pilings. I'd look up and see pigeons flying from one rafter to another or swooping in from the world beyond. I didn't have a relationship with pigeons back then, but those pigeons were intriguing and mysterious with their secret lives under the bridges.

My river trips gave me such joy, but the joy was pierced with sadness and longing, because I would never get to share them with the woman I loved.

(I'm sorry, but I have thought about interrupting these monologues ever since I started telling this story, and now I'm finally going to do it. For whatever reason, when I am dictating, every time I say "the woman I loved," the computer writes "the woman I love." My therapist would crucify me right now for mentioning it, but it seems significant.)

On one of my floats home from a particularly rough therapy session, I saw something poking out of the shallows, and I navigated toward it. It looked like a grocery cart but turned out to be a fancy mountain bike. So I lifted it up to give it a good look. The frame and the gears and the wheels were covered with bright-green algae.

That bright color reminded me of a toy I played with as a child, called "Slime." I'd sit on the corner of the living room couch while my family watched TV, my mother stretched out on the couch beside me. I would sometimes roll out the Slime like a baker making dough. I would sometimes stick it all over my fingers so that they looked like frog legs. And I would sometimes put it all over my face. As it oozed down and thinned out, it became somewhat translucent, and I could see my brother on the carpet and my father in his chair and my mother on her end of the couch, all laughing at me.

Because I have a mystery illness, it is easy to assign its origin to any strange thing that ever happened to me. Slime, and the toxic mask it made that I breathed through on weekend nights in the late 1970s while watching *Fantasy Island*, seems like a perfect candidate.

I pulled the slime-algae off the mountain bike and saw a tag fastened to the handlebar. The tag was a one-day pass from the previous day for a bike trail across the border in Idaho. How did a bike that was in Idaho the day before end up in the middle of a river in Missoula the next day? I imagined a motorhome, bikes strapped to the back, a happy family heading to their next destination, maybe Yellowstone or the Tetons, and then the strap that holds one of the bikes loosens, the bike falls off, maybe hits the bridge's railing, drops into the river, and drifts into the shallows.

I half dragged the bike down the river, half floated with it, until I got to the second bridge.

Years later, I would visit this same bridge nearly every day, standing under it with a bird on my head, a bird who I was secretly hoping would not release. I rolled the bike to shore, rested it against my hip, put on my shirt, and rolled the bike up the embankment. Then I rode home on it.

When I got to my little rented house, the garden blooming and the plum trees fruiting, I wheeled the bike to my shed. I called the police to let them know about it, and when no one claimed the bike, I held on to it. I didn't need a bike, but I fantasized that some opportunity would arise in which I could give it to the boy who had been in my life. Maybe he'd come back.

We hold on to things until there is nothing to do but let them go. Last summer, when I had to admit to myself that the boy would have outgrown the bike, I put an ad on Craigslist. Twenty-four hours later, it was gone.

———

EVERY FEW DAYS OR SO, I fill the shower stall with a few inches of cool water and I kneel on the bath mat, waiting for Two-Step to hop in. Once he's in the water, he leans to one side and lifts up his wing so that I can splash him under that wing and brush my fingers along his contour feathers. He alternates wings several times so I can thoroughly clean both sides. When he has had enough, he stops lifting his wings and does some furious flapping—his wings beat so hard that he actually lifts an inch or two off the surface of the shallow water and hovers

Buckbee & Fitzgerald

in midair. Then he hops out of the bath and leads me into the living room so he can find a quiet nook to dry off in. I love this ritual so much that sometimes I try to trick him into taking a bath (before he's ready for one) by running the shower faucet at a beguiling trickle. He's not easily influenced, but occasionally I'll hear his footsteps clicking across the kitchen tile and he'll poke his head into the bathroom, stride confidently toward me, and find his way to the water.

———

I HAD A POCKET FULL of screws when I learned that Brian 1.0 had died. They were brass screws of the Phillips-head variety, and there were forty of them in a soft plastic case. They had somehow evaded the pandemic supply-chain problem and made it to the stocked shelves of my local Ace Hardware store. When I checked out, I didn't want my penny back, I didn't want a bag, and I refused a receipt. I stuffed the screws in my coat pocket. The cashier asked for the rewards name, but I didn't give it to her, though I usually do, because the name belongs to the woman I loved, and that morning I couldn't summon the energy to say her name.

L. probably doesn't know it, but in the many years that have passed, I have spent a lot of time and money at that Ace, and she has accumulated quite a few rewards points. Sometimes I like to think that when she shops there and uses the points, she calculates how much money I have spent at Ace since her last visit, and maybe she gets to wondering what I am building or fixing or planting. My therapist tells me this is exactly the kind of thing—seven years later—I shouldn't be doing. (But I keep doing it anyway.)

I was buying the screws so I could put the boards together that would make Two-Step's nesting box, which is basically a three-sided window box with a couple of mousehole entrances. The box is now attached to the front of my house. Since it runs all the way along the top third of my living room window, I can see inside it. I just put the box up yesterday, but Two-Step and V. seem to be enjoying it so far. I haven't opened the mousehole doors yet, so the only way they can get in the box is from inside the house, when I open the window.

Next week I will open the mousehole doors, and Two-Step and V. will be able to fly from the house to the box to the yard outside. And then, a day or two later, I'll put some peanuts in my hand and Two-Step will fly across the living room and land on my wrist so he can peck at the peanuts and I'll lift him into the box. And he will then promptly start stamping around the way he does because he wants to be sure I know he owns everything. He will make his very loud, now very familiar, territorial trilling sound, and that will eventually encourage V. to join him in the box. And when she does, I will slide the window shut for the last time, and from then on Two-Step will never step foot in my house—the home he grew up in—ever again.

Sigh. This is hard to talk about. And I haven't even gotten to the part about my own death.

The good news is that for as long as Two-Step and V. decide to make that box their home, I will be able to see them through the window from my perch on the couch. And Two-Step will be able to look inside the house, and I like to think he will want to see me and maybe take one-tenth of the comfort from looking at me as I will from looking at him. Maybe once in a while I will stand up and raise my arm and press my hand against the glass, the way people visiting prisoners do in TV shows.

But what I really wanted to talk about was the phone call I got when I returned from the hardware store. I had those screws in my pocket when my disability lawyer called. I had been turned down for disability twice already, and I had my appeals hearing with an actual judge, but it was a hearing my lawyer assured me I was going to lose. People with chronic fatigue syndrome are rarely granted disability ("Chronically fatigued? We're all chronically fatigued. Get a job!"), and my judge in particular was a tough one. But what my lawyer said stunned me. She said, "The judge came back with a decision." My heart sank, and then she added, "She decided 'Fully Favorable.'" And what this meant was that in the court's mind there wasn't any doubt about the condition I was in. The judge's document ends, "The claimant has been disabled since Dec. 1, 2018."

And so, on that morning, nothing and everything changed. My health was the same as the day before, but now I was "disabled." The word, the designation, sat like a stone inside me. It was an inescapable weight, but it was also a weight lifted. I was not who I used to be, and I never would be again.

Of course, we don't stop being ourselves just because we become disabled. But for me, something had changed.

———

THESE DAYS, every day is a good day for Two-Step. When I open the door in the afternoon, he flies out, gliding over the birdcage that holds two broken-shouldered pigeons (a male and a female; neither will ever be able to fly again) that I've wheeled onto the porch, between the unkempt sprawling lilac and the ancient boxelder maple, over the low branches of the near plum trees and then the high branches of the far plum trees, and across the street to land on the pitched roof of my neighbor's house. He has so much force, he's not at all like the injured pigeon I found two years ago, a pigeon so frail, so vulnerable, so alone.

Sometimes when I am sitting with my beanie pulled down over my burning eyes, counting down the hours for a migraine to pass, I will hear Two-Step on the windowsill next to me, and

I will lift up the beanie and watch him looking out the window. If you just look at the golden eye apart from the rest of the bird, you might think it belonged to a Cooper's hawk or a horned owl; it is so intelligent, so keen, so fierce, so alert.

I guess it is evident that Two-Step and I have switched places. If he were my child, he would be taking care of me now. I'm glad he doesn't feel that responsibility, because I like him living his life. I like him zipping across the big blue sky on his way to the telephone wire that runs down the alley between Second and Third Streets, where he will meet up with his sweetheart, or craftily landing among a flock of pigeons on a rooftop and promptly proceeding to stamp his feet and turn in circles to show them who is in charge.

I have a migraine today, and I am thinking about how my friends might react when they hear I am "disabled." I have this image in my mind of a book being gently but decidedly closed. I am the book, of course, and my friends are the readers who may want a story with a little more action. This is not a rebuke, and I am not suggesting that my friends are prejudiced or unkind or anything. But if they want someone in their lives who is going to join them up at Lolo Pass on a clear winter's night to ski cross-country beneath the full moon, then I am not their person. If they want to grab hockey gear and toss it in the back of the truck and meet up at the rink to chase the puck, then I'm not their guy. Same goes if they want to sit in a movie theater, watching huge, bright images accompanied by a piercingly loud soundtrack. And so if they like those things—and who wouldn't?—I'm not their guy. If they like going out and having a few beers, I'm not their guy. If they like concerts or going for hikes or long walks, I'm not their guy. If they've reached a point in their lives where they have money and can travel, they're going to have to find somebody else. I've been lucky to have done all of these things for a long time, so I'm not complaining.

I'm trying to figure out how to say goodbye to Brian 1.0. I'm not there yet, but I think I know what the defining moment will be. Though it's embarrassing to admit, I'm just going to say it. The last cowardly bit of Brian 1.0 I'm holding on to is my profile on a dating app.

As with Facebook, I've basically never used the dating app I am on. A friend helped me with the technology, and it so happens that I set it up on the eve of the collapse of Brian 1.0. The photos are of me at the end of those days, on my second trip to Southeast Asia (a long and consequential trip that we'll go on together later in this story). My profile includes an anecdote about a sloth that fell from the forest canopy and almost landed on my head in a Costa Rican national park. I look at those pictures and I feel like I am looking at a different person, someone who had no idea he would soon be in a hospital bed in Kuala Lumpur, or that his carefree days of roaming the world were coming to an end. It is not a matter of changing the profile pics or the description—I need to take the whole thing down, bring out the wrecking ball and let it swing.

———

AS I SPEAK THESE WORDS, slow-motion spring continues here in western Montana. The cold front we're experiencing means I get a little more time with Two-Step before he moves perma- nently into the window box and I close the window on him and shut him out forever. My dictation routine will end then, too, and my story will be over.

At the end of December 2010, when I was about to turn forty-three, I took the first of my two extended trips to Southeast Asia. I was single and had completed my first adjunct-teaching semester at the University of Montana, where I was stationed in the office of a tenured English professor who was on sabbatical (fancy couches, ornate bookshelves). When I wasn't swimming sixty midmorning laps in the lap pool, I was playing hockey, so much hockey that I needed to sharpen my blades every other week (which is a lot for me). I had made some good friends (all of these friends, including L., were married), and we frequented Missoula's dive bars and fancy restaurants. I was lonely and hadn't dated anybody in Missoula in more than three years, and part of me thought it couldn't happen here. Since my brother had recently moved to Singapore, I had a perfect excuse for traveling, and I'd get to spend time with my nieces. My trip was scheduled to last at least six months, and maybe forever, but something happened, and I had to cut it short at five months.

My thirty-six-hour trip to Singapore began at dawn, when L. picked me up to take me to the airport. As I said, she was one of my good friends—for more than three years, she had leaned on me and I had leaned on her—and she insisted on driving me. It was frigid and dark in Missoula. The roads were empty and frost-covered. We could see our breath in the faint light of the car's stereo and the stream of streetlights. In the nine minutes it took to get to the airport, L. announced that since I saw her last—only a couple of days earlier—she had gotten separated. I felt such a sudden sense of disorientation that I almost asked, "Separated from who?" But of course I knew. I asked her why she was telling me this now, and she said it was something she thought I should know before I left Montana and started living half a world away from her.

———

MAYBE IT SOUNDS EXOTIC, romantic, and thrilling to travel the world alone. For some people, I'm sure it is all those things. (And only those things.) For me, it was also scary and lonely. I was afraid of eating the wrong food and being laid up sick as hell somewhere with gnats and rats and no air-conditioning. I talked to people on my travels, but I never joined, say, a group of Danes to suddenly go to Laos because there was going to be a great full-moon festival there.

What I wanted was to experience raw intensity. I'm not an adrenaline junkie, but I liked experiencing the world deeply. Like that midnight swim in Lake Michigan, for example, when I swam alone in the middle of the night through that glassy Great Lake toward the massive electric clouds filled with pink lightning.

I remember my brother was mad at me for not waking him up to join me on that swim in Lake Michigan. He loved doing things like that. And I would have enjoyed swimming in the middle of the night with my brother, but the truth is that with him there, I wouldn't have had the space to feel what I felt.

And that was the feeling Brian 1.0 was chasing when he decided to go to Asia.

I look back now and think how stupid I was. What a foolish Romantic. My therapist tries to reassure me that it was okay to develop that intensity-seeking "mode" as a child (probably as a response to some sort of trauma) and to continue it as an adult (because it had worked as a child), but now it has become "maladaptive." Because now I can't perform epic athletic feats. I can't travel to exotic lands. I have to accept—no, embrace—the less-than-ideal, whether it is in the world or in my head. This may not sound like much, but for me it will be harder than teaching a pigeon to fly.

———

YESTERDAY WAS MOTHER'S DAY, a special day, but something dreadful happened today—and I can't talk about it yet. So I'm going to talk about Two-Step and V. instead.

It was a special Mother's Day because V. finally laid an egg yesterday afternoon. Two-Step and I spent a good bit of the morning helping her reinforce their nest up on the shelf near the ceiling of my living room. The nest is made of twigs and twisty ties, and they kept sliding off the shelf. (The twisty ties seem to be their favorite nesting material.) Every time a twig or twisty tie fell, no matter where Two-Step was in the house, he would hear it hit the floor, and he'd promptly fly over to pick it up and bring it to V. She'd make pleasant cooing sounds and start arranging things all over again. On those rare occasions Two-Step didn't hear a twig or twisty tie when it fell, I'd be the one to pick it up, and I'd call him over and hand it to him. Since he doesn't like seeing me anywhere close to the nest, he'd fly at me prepared to do battle, but when he saw I was holding some nesting material, he'd take it from my pinched fingers with his beak and fly it up to V. Sometimes they do a little nest arranging together, side by side, moving in tight circles in the small space, and V. seems to like this, her wing feathers visibly trembling up and down (with pleasure, I think) when Two-Step moves a twig or twisty tie into place.

Mother's Day reminds me of my mother, of course, and I tried to remember her and how she was before the early dementia took hold of her.

Mother's Day also reminds me of conspiring to celebrate the woman I loved with the boy who also loved her. And this year it happened to be the seven-year anniversary of our breakup.

One time the three of us stopped at a mountain lake on the way home from a summer house we'd rented. We sat on the pebble shore to have a picnic and a few feet away from us a bat appeared and began to fly in erratic bug-catching circles. There was something odd about this bat putting on a show for us in the middle of the day. One of us—probably the boy—dubbed it "day-bat." And, for whatever reason, this was the funniest thing to all of us, so we kept working the term "day-bat" into our sentences. "Look at day-bat now." "Day-bat is back." "I think day-bat is the smartest because he gets all the mosquitoes to himself." That last one was the boy, and I'll never forget him saying it.

Part 3

(JULY–OCTOBER 2022)

IT IS JULY, AND IT HAS BEEN A LONG TIME SINCE I TOLD myself any of this story. Because of what happened right after Mother's Day, I couldn't follow the thread anymore. It wasn't writer's block, it was dread.

I couldn't talk about what happened and so I stopped talking to my computer and sending off missives one at a time to my editor. Two days turned into two weeks, which turned into two months. And I think I am only here now because my head is swimming and I am too disoriented to care. I got COVID a couple of weeks ago, and I am not sure what COVID does to people with my condition, and so I don't know if in a week or month or year I will be bedridden as a result of the Fourth of July barbecue I went to, which got rained out, which led to everyone gathering inside a super-spreading hot box of a house. I thought I had managed my symptoms of COVID, despite the medical system's inadequacy in keeping simple promises like returning phone calls and submitting prescriptions for antiviral packs, but then it came back with a punch a couple of days ago. My head is full of bees.

Last night, I waited until after what amounts to "rush hour" in these parts before venturing out to the pharmacy. The heat from the midsummer day was dissipating and it was refreshingly, terrifically windy. The treetops were swaying, and I was mesmerized by how tall the cottonwoods were, and how geometric, and how poetic the motion of the leaves was way up in the sky. There wasn't much traffic, and this was a good thing, because my fever seemed to be increasing by the minute and my head was pounding and my eyes felt like the balls in a pinball machine.

When my COVID came back, I felt scared and very alone and I reached out to the woman I loved to try to feel less alone, but I guess she is quite determined to not talk to me again, and when I looked up at those treetops I was thinking of her and wishing I had somebody I loved by my side who experienced as much joy and meaning looking at the trembling leaves on a cooling summer's night as I do.

My car windows were down, and the breeze was blowing, and I had a line from "Thunder Road" looping through my head that had been planted in my skull back when I was in middle school, when every night I listened to side one of *Born to Run* on the record player as I drifted off to sleep, telling myself those hero stories about saving the girl from a burning bus or making the dangerous game-saving play on the baseball diamond while she looked on, and my thick bedroom curtains would billow outward in the summer breeze and then get sucked inward, like they were breathing, while Springsteen sang, "Roy Orbison's singing for the lonely / Hey, that's me and I want you only," followed by the line that's haunted me ever since: "Don't turn me home again / I just can't face myself alone again."

And last night the song was circulating through me like toxic oxygen, over and over, as I navigated my way to the pharmacy, "Roy Orbison's singing for the lonely . . . Roy Orbison's singing for the lonely . . . Roy Orbison's singing for the lonely," and then quite suddenly I saw a big black bird dart out of the tall median grass—it looked more like a manta ray than a bird—and it swooped in front of my front bumper, and I didn't have time to react, and my foot didn't even touch the brakes.

———

I HAVE BRAIN FOG, and I really am not thinking so straight. After I hit the odd-looking bird, I pulled the car onto the shoulder and opened the door and stepped into the road. I don't know if I would say I was lucky I didn't get hit by a logging truck or a hippie on a scooter, but I don't think I looked to see if there were any oncoming vehicles. I was focused on confronting the grim truth of that dead creature, and I was worn down and feverish enough that I didn't really care what happened to me.

In my fevered state, I suddenly remembered a drive I took through eastern Nevada alongside the high desert of the Great Basin, its endless flatness stretching out as far as the eye can see. The two-lane highway belonged solely to me for many minutes at a stretch, and I was looking at the boundless flat land that used to be an ocean filled with sea creatures when a rather large ground bird flashed out of the broken stalks from the field to my right and I hit it going seventy miles an hour. When I pulled over to inspect the damage, my front grille was broken in half and there was so much carnage on the highway it would hurt me to describe it. Hitting an animal on a road trip can completely ruin you. I remember thinking, like I always did at times like that, what a shitty world it is, how shitty mankind is, how shitty I was, how we inflict so much damage on so many poor little creatures.

But last night, when I got out of my car to see the disaster I had caused, there was no blood. My fender wasn't broken or bent. There were no dents or marks anywhere, no sign that I'd hit anything at all. I wondered if I had imagined the bird altogether. I thought maybe something had blown out of the tall grass, like a piece of paper or a plastic bag. I looked around but didn't see anything. With my head spinning, I got back in the car and steered my bloodless vehicle onto the road and drove to the pharmacy and retrieved my medicine.

On the way home, all I could think about was that maybe-bird. When I got to the road where I had maybe-hit the helpless little thing, I did a U-turn and once again steered my car onto the shoulder. There was so little traffic I could just walk in the road, and I scanned the blacktop for evidence of a wounded animal. I thought maybe I'd spot him in one of the neighboring yards, hopping on one leg, and I could scoop him up and bring him home and maybe I could fix him up, or maybe he could just live with me forever.

I was bent over, zigzagging my way across the street, and seeing as I am skinny as all-get-out now, I knew I looked like one of those bedraggled men who walk the shoulders of our highways in tatters, lugging a giant cross. I searched for that bird, but I saw nothing—no hurt bird or once-bird, not even a stray feather— and before getting into my car, I gathered my senses, looked up, came out of my fever-fugue, and suddenly realized where I was standing. I was on the green grass in front of the house L. had moved into with her family of three when I first entered her life.

I don't feel comfortable talking about all this. This is someone else's private life, and it's not my story to tell. But I don't want my story to be incomplete, either. What you need to know is that in 2007, like me, L. and her family had moved back to Missoula after years away. But then she lost her only child—a three-year-old boy—to an accident. (The boy I would come to love would be born a year later.) Though I barely knew them, a mutual friend asked me to step in and help out where I could, and I said yes, not just to help my friend, and not just to help these people who were suffering loss, but as a gesture to honor the caretakers who had helped my mother so much as she was dying.

It was not too long after the accident when I visited L. and the boy's dad at a mountain lake north of Missoula. Tourist season had ended, and we canoed to a pebbly beach, where we were shrouded by the smoke of forest fires distant and near.

L. ventured into the shallows of the ice-cold knee-deep water and stood there for a long time, maybe thirty feet from shore. Eventually, I rolled up my pants and waded out to her. We didn't talk. What was there to say? After a while, she extended her arm and unfolded her fist. In her palm were five small stones, stones she had retrieved from the bottom of the lake, stones she said reminded her of her son.

She didn't say anything else, and we stood there in silence in the veil of smoke, in the very gentle swell of the water. Then she asked me to put my hand out, and I did, and she slid the five stones from her hand into mine.

I'm not so much the kind of person who comforts others by bringing them meals or by cleaning their homes. I did do those things, but that fall I found something else that seemed to help L. through the long hard days. At the time, I was working on an art installation, the centerpiece of which was a massive, model-railroad-style, miniature city that I was constructing in my kitchen. I asked her if she would like to build a skyscraper for the city from a model kit. This was clearly something she had never done before, and this particular kit contained a zillion pieces, each of which had to be carefully glued to the others in what was a near-Sisyphean task.

I told her she could come by my house anytime she wanted to work on her skyscraper, even if I wasn't home. She would sit on the floor in my living room, her back against the couch, working with all those pieces that were scattered across the coffee table. As the weeks went by, her building grew, one story at a time, until it was populated with tiny people and the penthouse was complete. She'd even found some miniature bears in my stash of model-railroad-scale critters and glued them inside a big corner office that had lots of glass windows. Despite everything she'd been through, L. couldn't help but be playful.

When the project was almost finished, I took those five little stones L. handed to me at the lake, and I dabbed them with glue and placed them throughout the miniature city. At that scale, they became boulders, and upon one of them, high on the bank of the city's sparkling river, I placed a small, boy-like figure who could sit there and marvel at the landscape and the wonders of his world.

And now, fifteen years later, I was at their house again, though they didn't live there anymore. I wiped the sweat off my feverish forehead (even though I wasn't hot) and I shivered (even though I wasn't cold). The grass was intensely green and the flowers were blooming and the wind was perfectly soothing and in the distance loomed the snow-peaked mountain where I used to go with L. We'd ski for hours and look for animal tracks and then lie on our backs in the fluffy snow, like children who are best friends, enjoying the winter wonderland without a care in the world.

I am rambling, I know, and I haven't even gotten close to the dreadful part. Even though my fever has come down a bit since last night, I'm still exhausted. I'm just going to keep talking into my computer, and I'm not going to worry about it making sense, and I'm not going to edit my words or even look at the screen.

———

I HAD AN EPIC DREAM last night. I've always told my fiction-writing students that including dreams in a short story is the lazy writer's cheap shortcut to creating character/conflict/meaning/ etc. But of course this isn't fiction, so it doesn't feel quite so cheap. (It still feels a little cheap.)

Right now I am dictating this on my couch under a blanket with my feet up on the coffee table, and a bird just stepped up onto the toes of my right foot and is perched there looking at me. I wouldn't say his look is "The Raven"–like, but it still feels like an indictment.

In the middle of this epic dream I find myself standing with L. in front of a large mirror. My back is to the mirror and L. is facing me. We are the ages we were when our life together got separated, and she asks, "What am I supposed to do?"

She is wearing a yellow sweater and she is putting on makeup, which is strange because she never wore much makeup, and I say, "You're supposed to be with me." She laughs because this sounds like a little joke, and in a way it is a little joke but at the same time it's not.

And she asks again, "*Really*, what am I supposed to do?" I don't know what exactly she is referring to and whatever it is seems unimportant, and so again I say, "You're supposed to be with me." And then I reach out and place the flat of my hand high on her chest, where I can feel the softness of her yellow sweater on my fingers, and the warmth radiating from her, and her beating heart, and I say, "I'm supposed to be with you."

Later in this jumbled dream, I'm in the back of a car and she's with me, and we're looking through the sunroof, the entire roof of the car is a sunroof, and the gray clouds are dissipating and a big round reddish moon appears and we stare at it, lying on our backs in that car, looking up at the sky, going who knows where.

When I got out of bed this morning, I remembered the dream, and then I remembered the first full moon I saw after my relationship with L. began to turn from a friendship of three years into something more.

The moon was turning toward fullness on the day L. dropped me off at the Missoula airport and I boarded the first of a series of flights that would take me to Singapore. The moon was waxing even more when I was in the Moscow airport and we messaged each other with Google Chat, our conversation no different from before, except that now we were talking about the sudden, enormous change in her life.

The moon became full when I made it to Phi Phi Island, an hourglass-shaped dot in the middle of the Andaman Sea, where my brother was vacationing with his family. This island had been wiped out by a tsunami in 2004, but it had been rebuilt. The resort side was hit by big waves, but the poorer side got hit by even bigger ones. Even though several thousand people died in the deluge, the island quickly got back to business so the tourists could slather on their coconut-scented sunscreen and complain about how long it took to get a mai tai.

One night after dinner I walked with my brother's family to the small white-sand beach along the bay. My two nieces were playing by the water and my brother and his wife sat in chairs and drank wine, and I sat a little apart, so I was with them and not at the same time. I heard the gentle giggling of my red-haired niece as she played peekaboo with a crab that was wondering if it was safe to come out of his hole. It was with her laughter in the background, the soft lapping sound of the waves hitting the shore, and the gentle rattle of the palm tree fronds swaying against each other that I glanced up and saw the moon. It looked a little like the moon in the movie *Joe Versus the Volcano* (a guilty pleasure of mine), way brighter than you'd think possible, and bigger, too, and I thought about how L. was under the same moon eight thousand miles away, and all of this together—the laughter, the crab, the breeze, the sunburn I'd gotten earlier that day, the salt air—made me feel like the day had turned into a wide-open doorway that I'd just stepped through.

When I got up this morning, I wondered how accurate this memory of mine was. I remember having had an email conversation with L. the next morning (her nighttime), so I decided to do a search in my email account. I combined terms like "crab" and "moon" and "niece" and was quickly directed to the conversation we had.

From our exchange I gathered that we had indeed been looking at a full moon. The full moon had coincided with the winter solstice, a rarity in and of itself, but in addition, and even more bizarrely, on her side of the world there had been a total lunar eclipse.

She wrote that the eclipse had turned the moon red. I didn't remember that. But I now wonder if certain memories from the other side of the doorway come alive when we dream. I just goo-gled the date of that lunar eclipse and the article confirms that, yes, indeed, L. was under a red moon and I was under a silver moon. The picture of the lunar-eclipse moon that accompanies the article looks exactly like the moon we saw from the back of the car in my dream last night.

The island rebuilt itself after the tsunami. Its scars don't show. Like the tide pool that is replenished with the coming tide, things can return to what they were. (Can't they?) Perhaps one day this headache will go away and Two-Step will be a fully wild bird again. And maybe I can make it to the other side of the world to sit beneath a full moon and listen to the palm fronds brushing up against each other, and the hole in me will be filled.

ABOUT A MONTH after L. told me her startling news about getting separated, I was staying in a remote place called Railay in Thailand. Because of its dramatic cliffs and rock formations, it was only accessible by boat. L. and I had been communicating even more than usual. Her life was changing dramatically, and at the very least I wanted to support her as best I could, even if it was from thousands of miles away.

At night, from the balcony of my second-floor bungalow, when the rain began and the fat drops plopped on the broad, firm leaves of the banana trees, I could hear the fruit bats rus-tling in their upside-down positions among the banana bunches or in the branches of the guava trees. I could sometimes catch the shadow or outline of a bat, but never much more than that. The thunderclaps echoed off the karst cliff walls, and the rain would pour, and it seemed the bats (which have the biggest hearts in proportion to their bodies of any mammal) were ecstatic to be out of their caves, in the dark of night, gorging on sweet, ripe fruit. Those enormous creatures had been flying around the skies like dragons for millions and millions of years, eons before anything like a knuckle-dragging human arrived on the scene.

It was hot in Railay. I'd strip down to my shorts and stand on the balcony in the rain until I cooled off, and then I'd go back in and respond to L.'s latest email. This is what friends do, especially best friends, and when you are in a faraway world, well, I guess it becomes easy to say too much.

I signed up for a night snorkeling boat tour because I wanted to see the bioluminescent plankton that rise from the depths of the deep, dark waters to feed off the dripping limestone cliffs.

The tour started in the late afternoon. As we headed to our first stop, we went past steep, rocky karsts that were covered with rigging. The rigging was used either to help in the collection of bird's nests or to deter the collection of bird's nests, I can't remember which. The takeaway for me was that some people really, really want to eat a soup made from a bird's nest. Some people think the birds that make those nests are swallows, but the nests are actually made by swifts. Swifts can fly for months without ever landing. They eat and sleep and have sex while in flight. The only time they spend on the ground is when they lay eggs and sit on them. Swift couples work together on child-rearing much like Two-Step and V. do. And it is the male swift who laboriously builds the nest—with his saliva. It takes him about a month or more to form a spit cup just big enough for his partner to lay some eggs in. (Yes, the nest that makes the soup is made of saliva.)

After our boat arrived at the tiny pink-sand island from where we would watch the sunset, I wandered down the beach to look for tide pools and wait for the sun to set over the Andaman Sea. I could see the surrounding islands' tall karst formations from the beach, and as I was standing there, bats—*thousands* of bats—started pouring out of them.

Apparently, the bats, which are called flying foxes, dwell in the safety of those remote crevices during the day, and at night they venture to the mainland to eat bananas in the pouring rain. What a world, I thought, as the vast, dark stream of bats went over me. I had no idea, of course, that those bats were the last thing I would see while I was still fully Brian 1.0. My journey to becoming someone else began on that spit of sand beneath those otherworldly creatures. And it started without me knowing, because one moment I felt like I had time-traveled to a prehistoric world, and the next I was unconscious, having fallen flat on my face.

I had never passed out before. In the movies, when people faint or pass out, it's a gentle process. Let's say a man hears a knock at the door, and when he opens it there is the woman he loved who has been gone for many, many years. The man's knees buckle a little, maybe he lifts his hand to his forehead, and he crumples to the floor slowly, maybe even gracefully. That is not how I passed out. I went down all at once. There was no swooning and no knee buckling and no arm groping for the support of a palm tree or some such thing. One second I was walking in my bare feet on the slight slope of the sandy beach, and the next I was trying—unsuccessfully—to get to my feet.

Something had happened, but I was too confused to know what it was. My brain was working about as well as my legs, which somehow got crossed every time I tried to stand up. I was vaguely aware of a group of people—three or four or six—running down the beach from maybe fifty yards away. I distinctly remember this one guy, in front of the rest, who was running very, very fast, and, despite the fog I was in, I found myself thinking, "Impressive." As he was charging toward me, he was yelling something, though I couldn't make out what it was until he got closer: "Don't touch your eyes!"

I must've been out for only a few seconds, and clearly, based upon how fast everyone was running, they'd all seen me go down. "Don't touch your eyes," this fellow, this hero, said again, and he put his hands on my shoulders and guided me into a sitting position. The thing is, I really wanted to touch my eyes. More than anything in the entire world what I wanted to do was ball my hands into fists and rub them back and forth across my eye sockets, because my eyes were itching like crazy. It turned out they were itching because when I passed out, I didn't close my eyes. That's how sudden and complete my temporary slip from this world was. I had fallen flat on my face without even blinking, and my eyes were covered with the sharp crystals of that coarse pink sand. I'm sure now, looking back, that if this man had not been so quick and so smart, I would've rubbed my eyes, which as far as I know would have made me go blind. But he got to me before I could touch them, and he asked for a water bottle from his friends and squirted water at my face, lightly brushing the sand away from around my eyes. "Oh boy," he kept saying to himself, as he continued to squirt water in my eyes and implored me not to blink. But the sand didn't seem to want to rinse out of my eyes. We went through a lot of water trying to get my eyes as clean as possible. But clearly, we only got part of the job done, because for the next few days, my eyes would occasionally "spit" sand out of that tiny hole at the edge of my bottom eyelid, making me feel pretty much like a lizard person.

I was disturbed by passing out like that, and I started thinking there was something very wrong with me. At the hospital in Singapore a couple of days later, the doctors asked me if I had been dehydrated or gotten sunstroke, and I said no and no. They could find no explanation for why I passed out. My heart was normal, the pictures of the inside of my head were normal, everything was normal. But I wasn't normal (though I felt pretty much normal). And subsequent events—more passing out, other neurological anomalies, and the eventual arrival of a particular kind of pain— would validate that something in me wasn't right. It would take years, seven to be exact, for my illness to be triggered for real, but that episode, beneath the bats, on the coarse pink sand, with the hero-stranger, was the start of something new.

I'm sure I told L. about the fainting episode, and as the weeks passed, I began to feel an increasing sense of urgency to get home. Walking the *sois* (alleys) of Bangkok, I felt the pull of home. Surfing in Bali, I felt the pull of home. Bicycling through rice fields and watching the Balinese ducks scatter, I felt the pull. In Singapore, in a high-rise with a wall of windows open to a coming storm, I felt the pull. And so, after five months away, I got back on a plane and flew to Moscow, then to Houston, and finally to my hometown airport, where the woman I had started to love was waiting to greet me.

———

IT IS TAKING LONG ENOUGH, isn't it, for me to finally get around to telling you about this dreadful thing that happened several months ago in May? Even though my COVID is gone and I have recovered from the fatigue, I am wiped out, in constant pain and anchored to the couch, and still completely unwilling to open up.

———

I WENT TO the foot doctor last week. When the doctor entered the examination room and took a look at my shin, she said, "Geez, what did you do to yourself?"

This question was prompted by the gash that was running from the middle of my shin toward my ankle, now covered with an oozy buildup of crusted blood. "Oh that," I said, "that's not why I'm here."

It just so happened that, the day before, a teetering step stool I was standing on in the yard fell out from under me, and I crashed

clumsily to the ground, injuring my shin. I was on the stool
because I was trying to plug a gap in Two-Step and V.'s nesting
box that a thieving squirrel had been squeezing through to get
at their food dish.

But my ankle problem started four months ago when I was
driving and I suddenly felt an intense lightning bolt of pain in
my left ankle, the ankle of my non-driving foot. It felt like there
was a miniature creature inside my ankle who had a car battery
and had decided to torture me with it. I was screaming when I
pulled off the road. Cars passed me by, maybe filled with people
who were going fly-fishing on the Blackfoot River to take advantage of the salmonfly hatch, or couples in love, who were taking
a blanket to a hillside where they could lie down and disappear
among the tall spring grass and yellow flowers, or maybe it was
L., who was driving past with her window rolled down. As the
warming spring air blew her hair back, did she hear the screaming of a madman?

Then the pain in my ankle went away as fast as it had come,
and I had no idea what else to do, so I eased my car back onto
the road and steered it in the direction of my couch.

It is important at this point to note that the foot that was
bothering me is not the same foot that bothered Two-Step. Mine
was the left one; his was the right. I wasn't trying to mirror his
pain or create a sympathetic injury, and in fact his foot had been
healed for so long that we didn't really think much about it anymore. For a few weeks I didn't feel the ankle pain, but then one
night in bed I got zapped again, and then again a couple of weeks
later, and I told my doctor that it had happened maybe fifteen
or twenty times total, though the recent lightning bolts were
less intense than the first few. She said I probably had a tendon
problem, but without an MRI we couldn't tell for sure. The thing
is, I couldn't afford an MRI, because becoming disabled meant
I had to be on Medicare, and when that happened I started my

deductible all over again. "What I really want to know," I asked the doctor, "is if I would do any permanent damage by doing nothing, taking no medical intervention."

"No," she said, "you just might feel some pain." She suggested I wear a brace, and she was happy and smiling the whole time, and I wondered what she thought of me. What was she seeing? I'm down to 135 pounds, and I was putting my bloody sock back on, and I was wearing my contraption-glasses the entire time, and my headache, which turns three and a half years old today (today!), was blasting away, and my face was likely contorted enough to make anyone want to keep their distance from me. Or maybe it is my desperateness for company, for companionship, that people recognize and that makes them want to turn away.

When I asked the doctor if it was normal for ankle tendon pain to be as sudden and intense as mine was, she looked at me quizzically and said, "No, that is kind of unusual."

When I asked her, "Is it unusual for the pain to come on when I'm not using the foot as opposed to when I'm using the foot?" she said, "Yes, that is unusual."

When I went to the neurologist and asked him if it's normal for a person to be woken up by a headache before dawn every morning, he said, "No, that is unusual." And when I did my colonoscopy and the prep failed to clean me out, I asked the gastroenterologist if that was normal, and he said, "No, that's pretty uncommon." When I went to a different neurologist and asked, "Is it unusual for someone without an underlying condition to have nighttime seizures that shake the bed so hard it wakes the beautiful woman you love sleeping next to you?" he said, "Yes, that is pretty strange." What is my stupid body doing to me? What is it trying to tell me?

People with fibromyalgia, which is a condition much like mine, also have problems with doctors. Their symptoms are often attributed to depression. People with Lyme disease can be mis-diagnosed as having multiple sclerosis, Bell's palsy, and even cardiac disease. And then there is Gulf War illness. In 2008 an investigative report ordered by Congress revealed that "Gulf War illness is real." But the soldiers they were referring to had developed rashes and headaches and episodes of brain fog and drooling after fighting in a war . . . in 1991!

I swear I'm not seeking attention or sympathy, but it seems as if my body is becoming irrelevant. My fantasies of saving the girl from the burning bus or diving into the ocean again with L. have been replaced with something much different now. The attainment of any of those things is so unimaginable that I can't even conjure up the fantasy. All I can fantasize about now is being "normal." I feel like I'm with Dorothy on the yellow brick road, on the way to see a magical person who I think will fix my broken self but who in reality doesn't exist. But I can't even be with Dorothy because I'm alone on the road. And I can't even be on the road because I don't have enough physical capacity, so instead I am anchored to my couch, adrift, waiting for my life to come back to me.

———

TWO-STEP LANDED on my head this morning! He hasn't been there since late last winter. I was standing outside and suddenly I felt this weight on my head that I immediately recognized as the exact weight of a pigeon, which brought back so many great memories, and all at once I didn't feel so alone anymore. It's crazy, isn't it? That a now-mostly-wild bird could make me feel so much better. Maybe doctors should keep birds in their offices and apply them like bandages to people in pain. It's as if Two-Step opened a kettle of loneliness inside me and released all the pressure. This took place a couple of hours ago, and though I'm sure the pressure is building up again, I don't feel it, I don't feel the aloneness.

———

YESTERDAY EVENING the lightning bolt in my ankle came back with a vengeance, and this time it wasn't a single bolt but a wicked storm. I sat on the couch screaming every five or ten minutes. And while I was doing this, I was also looking out the window because there was a pigeon in the yard, hanging around long after all the others had left. He was standing pretty still, and he had his head pulled down into his body, and his feathers were all puffed up, and I recognized this presentation from when Two-Step had the bout of salmonella poisoning a couple of years ago, back when I drove about 150 miles an hour to get him to the vet who saved his life.

And so there I was, on the couch, my foot on top of a pillow on top of the coffee table, glancing out the window from time to time to look at the ailing bird while I watched a TV show about two people in love in the mid-'80s who experience intensity together, accompanied by a soundtrack of the music I grew up with—by bands like Echo and the Bunnymen, Roxy Music, and especially New Order. Foot, window, TV; foot, window, TV; foot, window, TV. I was on the emotion carousel, going round and round.

I miss being looked at by a beautiful woman the way the woman in the show looks at her boyfriend. I can't imagine being looked at by anyone that way now. How could I ever return the kind of intensity I admire and desire in a partner when I can't swim out to the reef, or fly to a remote island, or step on the ice in my hockey gear and chase kids half my age who have played hockey twice as long as I have all around the rink? I can't even stand in front of a classroom of college students and lead them all at once into a clearing where their minds have never been before.

It was almost dark outside and that sick bird in the yard had moved and I couldn't see him anymore. I figured he found cover somewhere, and that's all well and good except for how wise owls are. And how raccoons are renowned bandits (they steal pigeons). And cats, well, there is a common expression about how curious they are. Any one of those monstrous denizens of the night is cataclysmic to a stricken bird. So I decided to go look for where the pigeon was hiding, so that I could scoop him up and bring him safely into my house (aka pigeon coop).

I looked under the rosebushes and along the fence line and in the gap between the house and shed, but I didn't find the pigeon. But when I hopped back to my porch, there he was, pressed up tight against my door. He was alert enough to be scared, and before I could push the door open and guide him inside, he half flew, half walked away and settled beneath the lilac bush.

Pigeons have awful night vision, which is why you don't see them flying around the city after dark. I can't understand why their night vision is so poor. After thirty million years, wouldn't their vision have improved? Then again, maybe evolution kept their eyes bad, saddled them with this supposed disability, so as to force them to hunker down in the night where they could steer clear of those monsters I was talking about, the ones with the claws and teeth and talons.

I decided to let him be until it was pitch-dark, and then I'd crow-hop out of the house and grab him. I retreated to my couch and put my foot up and watched that beautiful woman who reminded me of L. on TV. An hour or so later, I hopped over to where my headlamp was, strapped it on, and hopped to the kitchen. I opened the door and slid my good foot forward across the doorjamb so as to find steady purchase, and my toe kicked something that was resting on my porch. It felt like a popcorn ball. I shone my headlight down and it wasn't popcorn but rather the sick bird, and now he was rushing away, as best he could, like a car thief dodging the spotlight of the police helicopter. Whenever he escaped the beam of my headlamp, I lost track of him, but he couldn't go far and then I'd catch him in the light again. The pain in my ankle started zapping, and I was terrified that I would hop on top of the bird, and I chased him in and out of the light until I finally cornered him behind my propped-open screen door. Then I bent down and gathered him up.

Pigeons are big birds, but they're surprisingly light, and they are soft and warm and they don't resist if you hold them tight. I carried him inside and brought him into my spare room and set him in a box that was poked with holes. Other birds had triaged in that same box. I put a comfy towel in one corner and some water and a sprinkling of food in another and I left him in peace.

A thought was nagging at me, and is still nagging at me, and that is, why, of all places, did this pigeon choose to wait out the night right up against my door? It's not a warm or sheltered place. I'd noticed he was a classic rock pigeon, gray with two wide black bars that wrapped around his lower body—and Two-Step and V. had a baby this winter that looked like him. Was this the same bird? Was this Two-Step's progeny? Was he trying to get back to where he knew it was safe, where he was born, where he grew up? I don't know for sure, but I think it was him. It seems as if the pigeons that are born in the house or the hutches linger longer in the yard than the other pigeons. I think they are comfortable and feel safe there because, to them, it is home.

In the box in my spare room with the door closed, Popcorn had warm shelter and as much nourishment as he wanted and all he was missing was some companionship. Isolating Popcorn like that made me think of the countless people who've had to die alone during the pandemic, and what a difference it would have made if they could have been in the company of others. My poor aunt, for instance. She lost the love of her life that way. I was tempted to move Popcorn into the room with my other injured birds (aka my kitchen), but I worried that maybe he had a communicable disease, and I'd end up killing them all.

———

DID YOU KNOW that many cities and towns kill pigeons? They even make laws that allow citizens to kill them. I try to imagine a board of elected officials gathered around a big oak table: "All in favor of killing the pigeons?" And then a loud collective "Yea," followed by a quiet single "Nay."

In fact, the pigeon is one of three birds that have no animal rights protections, the other two being the house sparrow and the starling. The difference between the latter two and the pigeon is that we domesticated the pigeon in the first place. The reason pigeons are hanging around populated areas is because we taught them to do so. Their only mistake was letting themselves get close to us. It's easy to make that mistake. And for the crime of allowing themselves to be domesticated, pigeons are shot and trapped and poisoned and collected for sport so falconers can release them and watch their pet hawks or falcons or eagles tear them apart in midair.

If you were to read the web page about pigeons on the Montana Fish, Wildlife & Parks website, you would think the pigeon is equivalent to a bubonic-plague-carrying alien-zombie rat. Oh, the horrible damage pigeons do to our society! They defecate on cars and porches and patio furniture and ruin everything! And the diseases! So many diseases! All those impossible-to-pronounce Latin names mean they must be really bad. And this is Montana, a place known for its *love* of wildlife, with few urban areas and not a lot of pigeons. The web page is titled "Living with Pigeons," but all it talks about is how to kill them.

This is not to say that the pigeon is entirely harmless. But, hell, dogs carry as many diseases, and cats, too. The best advice to follow is from the CDC. And this part is true—they actually put it out in a press release—people should not "kiss or snuggle" their backyard poultry. This became necessary during the pandemic, when housebound people began raising chickens for their eggs. The problem was, those same people were lonely. All across the country, while the virus milled about, people were falling in love with their roosters and hens.

———

I GOT ENGAGED on today's date eight years ago. I remember my sense of finally having arrived at a meaningful place in life.

I know what my friends are thinking. They are thinking, "Eight years? Get over it!" And maybe I would if I could understand what happened. Maybe I would if I hadn't spent the last four years in constant pain. I miss L. I miss comfort and hope.

Doctors say I am depressed. "Well, of course I'm depressed," I tell them. "I've had a headache for three and a half years. How would you feel?"

Because I weigh 135 pounds, the doctors ask me if I am eating. "As much as I can," I tell them. The problem is, I am almost always nauseous, and eating only makes me feel worse.

I have a new therapist. A second therapist. She is called a "pain reprocessing therapist." At our last meeting, she asked me why I wanted to be in pain. She said that everyone she has worked with wants to be in pain for some reason (even if they are not fully aware of it). Maybe it means they can work less or will get more attention from others, or perhaps it's a form of penance for some past transgression. I thought about her question for a long time and said, "I can't think of a single reason I want to be in pain." At our next meeting she said she spent the week thinking about it, and she couldn't think of a reason, either.

I DO UNDERSTAND, I guess, why so many people think of pigeons as pests (or don't think of them at all). We have been conditioned to think of certain animals as threats that can and should be removed. We need to exert control over our animals and our lands and our homes. "Who cares," people say, "they're just pigeons." Yes, they are "just" pigeons. And they have been flying in choreographed precision in flocks of twenty or thirty or fifty or more, over land without buildings, without roads, without sidewalks, benches, trash cans, and the other things of man for millions of years. And "just" one of them saved my life.

The Montana Fish, Wildlife & Parks website fails to mention that the best way to control the pigeon population is to get rid of people like me. I have been feeding a flock of pigeons ever since Two-Step's offspring left the house. Over time, more and more pigeons have shown up. I don't know how to feed Two-Step's kids and the other birds I have rescued and released without feeding them all. I now have thirty or forty pigeons visiting my yard twice a day. And there are other people around town who are doing the same thing. Instead of trapping and euthanizing and poisoning and shooting these creatures, the best thing Fish and Wildlife could do is make two dozen phone calls telling us idiot pigeon-feeders to stop what we're doing. I'm pretty sure that every pigeon feeder would step away from their seeds if they learned that the city was otherwise going to start poisoning their beloved pigeons. I'm trying to slowly taper the amount of food I feed the flock, but it is hard to deprive them of such a basic need. In my stricken state, I find it impossible not to feed the little guys and to allow nature to take its course, the course that requires the small and the sick, the most vulnerable, to die first.

I don't know what made Popcorn sick. It is possible that my town at some point passed an ordinance that allows them to kill as many pigeons as they want. I heard from another pigeon enthusiast that our town has done this on occasion. The poison most often used to "cull" (aka kill) pigeons is called Avitrol. The poison is mixed into grain and fed to the birds. After ingesting it, the pigeon's nervous system gets attacked. Basically, the birds begin having seizures (just like I have) and they develop other neurological problems (just like I have) and then they die.

Of course, Popcorn wasn't displaying those kinds of neurological symptoms. He looked lethargic more than anything else, the way Two-Step did when he had salmonella. But there is a second poison that some towns use, and this poison works by slowly shutting down the bird's organs. That's what Popcorn looked like whenever I checked on him.

The next morning, I had to get up at an ungodly early hour—it was still dark outside—to get ready to go to the hospital for a ketamine treatment. All my treatments are at medical facilities because the dose they give to people with chronic pain is massive. Before I left I checked on Popcorn. I collected the things I would need while in the land of ketamine—the soft knitted beanie L. made for me, the zip-up fleece my niece got me because its color is "pigeon blue," and the high-end over-the-ear headphones my brother gave me.

The last thing I did before I went to meet the Uber that was to take me to the hospital was check on Popcorn again. I peered into his box and he was lying on his side, and though he was breathing, they were slow, shallow breaths. His eye looked up at me and I wanted to tell him something comforting. I wanted to pick him up and hold him so he wouldn't feel alone. I realized that talking or holding would scare him more, and the best thing I could do for him was to turn out the light, cover his box, and close the door.

That was hard to say. I'm a mess right now. I'm not sure if weeping will come out on dictation, but it should.

———

A FRIEND ESCORTED me home from my ketamine treatment and helped me stumble into bed. I slept most of that day and night, and the next morning the first thing I did was go to my shed and find a soft, thick cloth. I picked up Popcorn and carefully wrapped him in it. Then I went outside and placed his body in a hole I had dug weeks earlier (in Montana, you have to prepare for the worst before the ground freezes), and I buried him.

I really do get it. I get why not everyone is a fan of the pigeon. But it is impossible to hold one of these birds in the palm of your hand and not protect it with all your life.

———

WHILE I WAS in my ketamine fugue, I experienced birdness. I didn't become a bird, but when I saw a glimpse of pigeon silhouettes against a midnight-blue sky, I became part of it all, the near-infinity of flocks that have been flying against the same-colored backdrop for countless generations.

I thought about those fish, too, those fish in the tide pools, the ones that are identical copies of their bigger siblings who are swimming out in the open ocean, above and around and through the ancient corals. The tiny Moorish idols in the tide pool had the same long, streaming dorsal fin and the same black-and-yellow hues as the ones the woman I loved and I snorkeled with at places like Puako and Kealakekua (also known as Captain Cook) and Two Step Bay. Some people think of the Moorish idol as a symbol of happiness, and when L. and I were surrounded by schools of them I was quite sure those people were right.

THE PROTOCOL for using ketamine to treat pain is different from its other applications. Such a huge dose of the drug is given that it has to be administered through an IV in a highly supervised medical setting, and the result is essentially paralysis. (Waivers about accidental death are signed right before the drip begins.) The dose is dripped over a long period—three-plus hours. And so that means I am lying propped up in a bed in the very position the neurologist recommended a long time ago. Occasionally, I experience a strange sensation in which my lower arms feel like they have been inflated to preposterous proportions, a phenomenon my nurse referred to as "hot-dog arms."

None of this is remotely unpleasant, mind you. I am under lots of warm blankets, I have the over-the-ear headphones that my brother gave me for my birthday over my earplugged ears, and I am listening to nature sounds—tide pools filling, thunder clapping. I wear an eye mask to block out the already dim lights. (Though I have learned this isn't even enough, and sometimes during my infusion I will call out, "Bright lights!" as if I am a gremlin. The nurses—they are very caring and feel even more so while I am in "K-land"—have learned to put large gauze pads over my eyes and then tape them down so no light at all can peek through. This seemingly small act of kindness makes an enormous difference in my experience.)

No matter how out of it I am on ketamine, I am somehow always able to picture the scene exactly as it is as I lie semi-comatose, propped up in the hospital bed. In my mind I can see the blood pressure cuff on my right arm, inflating and deflating every few minutes. I can see the IV line needled into the forearm of my left arm. I can see the zippers pulled down on my hoodie and the vest my niece gave me and the five glued-on heart monitor pads across my chest. I can see myself mouthing the one-word chorus to the Beatles song "All You Need Is Love," and sometimes even mumbling out loud. (*Love, love, love. Love, love, love.*) And in the picture—every time—is my teddy bear (the one L. gave me). I bring him to all my infusions (four so far), and just before the drip starts, I prop him up between my slightly spread legs over the warm white blankets the nurses have draped over me, so he is facing me, and I get to imagine him like that the entire time (even though by the time I "wake up" several hours later, and I slowly get comfortable enough with the idea of having the tape on the gauze pads removed, then a bit later the gauze pads removed, and then a bit later the eye mask removed, and then a bit later my eyelids "removed," i.e., opened, the teddy bear has toppled over).

In my own bed, at nighttime, when I am in that propped-up position and I have the teddy bear lying on my chest, it helps me remember the ketamine experience and reconnect to what my Buddhist mentor calls "the mother ship," which is the massive marvel that reveals itself in my ketamine infusion experience, and through some yet-unexplained neurological process, by reenacting the posture and the setting as best I can, my physical pain is reduced and I somehow feel calm and I somehow feel loved.

———

RECENT STUDIES CONCLUDE that although less than 5 percent of adults with chronic fatigue syndrome will recover, around 50 percent of adults will improve over time. (I don't seem to be on that trajectory.) But the term "improve" is misleading, because—to me, at least—it seems to suggest measurable improvement. I think most chronic fatigue sufferers who "improve" do so modestly, and most of that can be attributed to accepting their illness and limiting their exertion. The recovery rates are not much better for people with fibromyalgia or Lyme disease or Gulf War illness.

I'm not the person I used to be. And I'm proving to be a horrible Buddhist because I am resisting becoming the new person I'm supposed to be. I fight this illness, though doing so makes me sicker, and that makes me feel worse, and so I resist even more. I suppose this is the definition of a downward spiral.

The high-dose ketamine infusions are intended to relieve my pain, and I do think they are helping. During those three hours of mind-altering paralysis, I can only manage to speak a few recognizable words, but in every one of my four infusions, I have said at some point, "Come back to me." The great thing about ketamine—or one of the great things—is that I am saying these words because I believe I can will what I say into being.

Last winter, when I posted pieces of this story on Facebook, I began hearing from high school friends, including some I haven't been in touch with for decades. I talked to one of them on the telephone, just like we used to for hours at a time a zillion years ago. She told me she had been out to lunch with the old gang and they'd started talking about my Facebook posts. I didn't think much about it at the time, but now I'm wondering why. Why were they talking about me? I think something about what I said in my Facebook posts made them worried I was on the verge of some kind of self-harm.

I suppose if you looked through my window last winter, what you would have seen might have been concerning. I was a very thin, pale man with an overgrown beard and the equivalent of a small flock of wild birds perched around me at all times, and everything in my tiny house was covered in bird-dropping-stained sheets. But that wasn't really me, or at least it wasn't the me I used to be.

I'm in a bad mood. A week out from my ketamine infusion, I'm realizing that the wonder-glow isn't going to stick. The person I was on the "trip" was the person I used to be, and now I am drifting toward the person I am going to become.

———

WHEN I WAS five years old, my family followed my father's Icarus-like career from New York to the suburbs of Chicago. Previously, he'd been a detective, and then he'd taken a high-level, somewhat mysterious job at an international security company, and now he'd become a regional manager at that same company. (He wouldn't be flying on secretive assignments around the world to places like Colombia and Cuba anymore.)

I used to think my family was normal. My parents attended their kids' sporting events and school functions, my dad coached baseball a few times, and my parents hosted and went to neighborhood gatherings. Shortly after my father took the regional manager job, he got embroiled in some kind of office politics and decided to quit and become an independent steel broker. His job entailed taking calls from companies that needed oddball orders of steel and then he'd track down the steel, from which he would make a commission. His office was our kitchen table; his technology was a typewriter, a second phone line, and a yellow legal pad; and he adopted a pseudonym (for some reason) which was Joe St. John (for some reason). I wasn't allowed to touch that phone, but sometimes he had me answer it, and on those occasions I was instructed to say, "Joe St. John's office."

I don't know why things changed, but my parents pretty much stopped going out, they almost never had anyone over, and our family of four became increasingly isolated.

Since my father wasn't leaving the house, he felt no need to dress for work, and he conducted his business at the kitchen table in ratty boxer shorts and his old fraternity sweatshirt, which looked even worse for the wear because he was constantly sucking on the collar. He did crossword puzzles and watched soap operas, smoked a ton of cigarettes, and when it got close to five o'clock, he would start having his sons shuttle vodka martinis from the kitchen (where my mom made them) to his chair in the living room.

Around that time, when I was eleven or so, my very quiet, almost mouselike mother returned to her job as a nurse. That my mother could work a job, *had* worked a job before I was around, kind of stunned me. I thought her job was taking care of me, but apparently other people needed her, too. She worked at an assisted living facility, where she helped old and severely disabled people. I'm quite sure that the people in her care felt deeply cared for, as I always did, as did all the injured birds and bunnies and other creatures that came across her path.

My father became a recluse. Some nights he would sleep outside on the patio in a strappy lawn chair. Sometimes before going to bed I'd lie in the chair next to his and we'd stare silently up at the stars. At some point I'd get up and go to bed, and sometimes when I came downstairs the next morning he'd still be out there.

MY FATHER AND I used to write humorous poems to share with each other. Though he had been a literature major in college, I think his career had been guided by the wishes of his own father, who expected him to become a corporate man. But in his free time, my father enjoyed writing the sort of clever poem that could make a twelve-year-old boy (i.e., me) laugh, and when I came downstairs in the mornings, I would often find one of his poems scribbled on a scrap of paper stuck to the refrigerator. I always felt special when I saw that scrap of paper, and I always felt excited about responding with my own clever poem, which would make him laugh and make him want to keep the game going.

When I was in seventh grade, I wrote a poem for school that stirred up a controversy. I didn't intend for it to be controversial, and I don't remember the lines that well, but it was about a boy walking in the woods with his beloved companion. As the two venture deeper into the woods, the mood gets more intimate—they look into each other's eyes, they brush up against each other, that sort of thing. The last stanza offers a climax of sorts. And this part of the poem I do remember:

He reached into his pants
And out he took his toy.

My teacher was furious. I don't think she found it very amusing that one of her students was writing a poem about a "toy" in his pants. She gave the poem an F and wrote a scathing comment in red pen at the top. Apparently, it made no difference to her that the last two lines of the poem were:

He gently tossed it to his dog
And his world was full of joy.

When I showed the poem to my father, *he* became furious—at my teacher. He marveled at the way I led the reader through the stanzas to assume that the boy's companion was a girl, even though I never used the word "girl," and the lines were ambiguous enough to suggest that the companion could actually be a dog (which it was, based on my beloved dog Max). I had used the same playful language my father and I used in our poems, and he was indignant. He loved the poem. "Screw her," he said and stuck it on the refrigerator.

BEFORE I VISITED my father for the first time at the hospital, I stopped at a grocery store and bought a five-pound bag of flour. He was propped up in his hospital bed when I presented it to him. I told him I had thought about getting him a bouquet of "flowers," but instead decided to get him one "flour." My little joke (I know, not a very good one) brought him joy. He plopped that bag of flour down on his tray table, and every time a hospital worker entered the room, he would say, "Look what my son brought me." The workers didn't understand the joke, but that made not a lick of difference to my father. He was on the verge of death and he was beaming at me.

One of the biggest gifts my father gave me was staying alive for several years after he got sick. I wish it had been longer, but it was enough time for us to reconcile and become friends again. But I now recognize that the even bigger gift my father gave me was his dying, which freed me from the burden of his expectations. Because of him, I'd always felt compelled to pursue conventional success, fruitlessly working at jobs that didn't suit me, but after he was gone, I heeded the call to a different sort of life, which eventually led me to the wilds of Montana.

———

I WENT TO HAWAII seven times with L. Each time we snorkeled the coves, chased the Moorish idols, and watched the stars against the black blanket of night. We were always disappointed when we had to leave, so at the Kona airport, before we boarded our flight home, we would ease our sadness by booking our next trip. On our second-to-last visit to the Big Island, in 2014, I proposed to her on a sandy beach on the Kohala Coast even though by then we had already decided to get married. After she said yes, as if the ancient Hawaiian gods were sending us some sort of prophetic, albeit curious, message, a naked Hawaiian fisherman appeared on the rocks beside us. He paid no attention to us as he gracefully cast his line far out into the ocean, hoping to catch a snapper or bonefish or ladyfish. When the woman I loved and I got home to Missoula, we signed the papers for our new house and I helped her and the boy move in, gave notice to my landlord, and we began planning our wedding ceremony and honeymoon, both of which would take place on the Big Island.

L. was a water creature, too, and swimming in the ocean as well as in rivers and lakes became a sacred rite for us. We called it a purification ritual. We even did it when we were apart as a way of feeling close, a gesture that meant our love was sacred.

One time we were snorkeling in Puako Bay, not far from the place where Two-Step gets his name. We had the water mostly to ourselves, and we followed each other in the shallows, pointing at corals and butterfly fish and Picasso triggerfish, and then we swam out far from shore, where we'd have the entire ocean to ourselves.

At one point she dipped below the surface and vanished. When she finally came back up, she was excited about something. She pushed her snorkel to the side of her mouth and raised the mask to her forehead. I couldn't imagine what she might have seen, especially since the bottom of the ocean was way too far below for either of us to reach. "Just go down," she said. "Fifteen feet, then wait." So I dove down, pinching my nostrils and blowing the pressure out of my ears, and as I went farther, the water became colder, darker, more mysterious. I didn't notice anything unusual. But then I heard something. It was high-pitched and sort of melodic, and though I'd never heard it before, I immediately knew what it was. It was the sound whales make when they are singing to each other.

When I surfaced, L. was treading water, waiting for me, and she was smiling, maybe more than before. I was smiling, too, because the whales were beautiful, and so was she.

Buckbee & Fitzgerald

This was one of those moments when it felt like a door was swinging open. Sometimes L. opened the door for me, and sometimes I opened the door for her. Going through the door takes you into an endless world of wonder. I feel like I have been chasing that door my whole life. There are not many people who can open that door for me. But L. could.

———

THE FIRST MOVIE I watched with L. was *Joe Versus the Volcano*. She knew I liked the movie and was curious about it, so one night we got comfortable in a bed that was way too small for the two of us and ordered it up. In the middle of the movie, there is a scene in which the eventual "soulmates" (ugh, I know), played by Tom Hanks (Joe) and Meg Ryan (Patricia), are adrift in the ocean, floating on the flotsam of a shipwreck, Joe's steamer trunks. Exhausted and sunstroked, perhaps delirious, the character played by Tom Hanks watches the moon rise above the glowing, gently rippling sea. The moon is cartoonishly huge in this scene, and intensely bright, and Joe looks at it in awe and falls to his knees while praying, thanking God for his life, and he starts to say, "I forgot how big—" just before he passes out.

L. loved the moon. It had some special meaning for her, kind of like it did for Joe in that scene, like it did for me in that dream I told you about. Now, whenever I see the moon, I feel a great sense of awe and love for the vast universe, and for L., too.

In the many years since L. disappeared from my life, my therapist has asked me repeatedly what it was about her, and I have always failed to find the words that could explain it. I think my therapist thinks my idea of love is immature. Like my longing for intensity, she calls it maladaptive. But as I change into this other person (Brian 2.0), as I get sicker and sicker, thinner and thinner—as I get closer to disappearing—I don't want to give up on this crucial part of who I am/was. I don't want to let go of my definition of love, and why deep love, love with "the one," is so important. I want to believe that there is a door-opener out there for me, and nothing in the world matters more than the most important assignment we get in life, which is opening those doors (to the wonders of the natural world and the universe). To me, seeking love like this is a virtue, just like seeking to be loyal, honest, or kind to others are virtues.

My therapist, sitting in the chair in her little office while I sit on the couch, has asked me over and over why there are so few people who can be "the one" for me. She has also asked why a person would need "the one" to begin with. I mean, why be so demanding?

It may be stupid, and it may be immature, and it may be maladaptive to write this way about someone who in the end couldn't or wouldn't have me, and who made the choice to vanish from my life. But I think that love is enormous, like Joe's moon, and transcends everything, contains everything, and because of it, all can be understood and all can be forgiven.

In this illness, with all its pain and aloneness, with pigeons flying all over the place, I don't ever want what happened to Joe to happen to me. I don't ever want to forget, even for a second, how big it all is.

I think that when I'm on my deathbed, whether that is this year or the next, or twenty years from now, what I will want is for L. to reappear so I can tell her all this. The petty things that were said or done, honestly, what difference do they make? I hope she has come to see in herself what I saw in her. I want her to be happy, even—or especially—if the life she chose is not so ideal. No matter where you find yourself, there are always more doors to open. Two-Step has taught me that.

I SUPPOSE THE REASON I am avoiding the dreadful thing is because to tell you about the dreadful thing I have to tell myself about it, late at night in my bed in the dark, and I really don't want to do that. But I will try.

This past winter, as the pandemic continued to isolate us all and turn us into recluses (not by choice, like my father), I felt my aloneness. Of course, Two-Step helped me feel less alone. And so did the six or eight or ten other birds that were flying or marching around my increasingly feather-strewn house. But by the time spring rolled around, most of them (including Two-Step and V.) were spending the entire day outside. Of the two juveniles from Two-Step and V.'s final winter brood, the older one returned to the house late in the evening, but he, too, spent almost all day outside. And then he stopped coming inside, and I would only see him from time to time under the lilac bush with a handful of other pigeons, learning how to be a real bird.

Of course, I still had the two broken-shouldered pigeons who lived in the cage (and the babies they were having), but they spent most of the day outside as well because I rolled their cage onto the porch each morning. From time to time I'd go out to the porch and open the lower door of their two-story cage so they could hop out and venture around, doing some mingling of their own. The male in particular liked to go out. He'd wander through the remnants of last year's perennial garden looking for a twig, then waddle quickly back to the porch, hop into the cage, and give it to his partner, and then he'd repeat it all over again. I'd give him a long recess until my anxiety about hawks got too great for me and I'd reluctantly usher them back into their cage and close the door on them.

By then I had released the ring-necked dove, the one who used to sit on the bookcase behind me exuding peacefulness and calm, and I'd see him stop by from time to time, usually in the thinning light of late evening, after the pigeons were gone, so he could forage in peace for little bugs and dirt and whatever else he needed.

And then there was one. Just one bird who would spend the majority of the day in the house with me. This was the younger of the two juveniles, Two-Step's other baby. He was different from every other pigeon I ever had flying around my house. He would go outside in the morning, but he wouldn't stay long. Because it was spring and pre-housefly season, I'd often leave the door open, and he'd come in when he was ready. Eventually, I had to keep the door closed, because one day I looked up from my couch and there were about twenty pigeons in my kitchen, pecking at the floor for the seeds that the caged birds were constantly scattering all over the place. After that, I would frequently get up and open the door and the little pigeon would come in after a minute or two.

What he liked to do more than anything was sit on the windowsill next to the couch and look out the window at the other birds (and whatever else birds like looking at). He never got jittery or frightened when I got up and moved around. He seemed to feel totally safe with me. And that was comforting.

It's crazy, isn't it? That a little, nameless, mostly wild, soon-to-be-released (maybe?) bird can do that for you?

From where I sat, on the increasingly indented rut in the corner of my couch, with my headache pounding away, that stupid coronavirus evolved-and-run-amok all over again, my knit hat pulled down over my eyes, that pigeon was no more than an arm's length away. Occasionally, I would roll up the hat and look out the window, check on the birds who were milling about beneath the lilac bush, and then I would look at him on the sill and he would look back at me. He seemed utterly content and at peace, and we would look out the window together while the hours passed.

I felt so connected to this little bird. He had such a positive and curious personality. He was a door-opener, there was no doubt about that, because when I saw him looking out the window, I'd look, too, and I'd feel some relief from the stress and pain and hopelessness because I'd be reminded how interesting the world is, how if you can just be calm and curious, you might experience its beauty and wonder with a like-minded creature. Look, the flowers on the lilac bush are coming out! And do you see that pigeon over there with one wing stretched out wide in the sun so that he can get a dose of vitamin D? And the other pigeon in the birdbath shaking water like drops of diamonds from his wings?

The little pigeon had the generic-pigeon appearance of his parents (no offense, Two-Step), with one exception—his legs and feet were mostly black. (Many pigeons have pink or even red legs and feet that are covered with white feathers so it looks as if they are wearing leg warmers.) He was "just" a pigeon, but when he sat on the sill as we passed those long spring days, he helped me feel a lot less lonely. I feel kind of ridiculous saying that a bird can make me feel that way. But I'm not who I was, and who I am now can say it, maybe needs to say it, because who I am now needs a bird like him on that sill.

———

I'M SORRY, but I can't keep talking about the dreadful thing. Life seems so precious to me now, so vulnerable, and it's hard to tell this part of the story. I guess I will have to get back to it later.

I rented a big house on a big lake with L. one summer. It was several years after she'd gotten separated and almost several years after we'd gotten together. Her family visited us—her mom and stepdad, her stepsister and two of her stepsister's children. To me, having grown up in the house of a recluse, this seemed like a hive of activity. Two kids playing a game of Trouble over there, a man drinking coffee out on the dock, and on the porch a child, L.'s child, building a 3D model of the Tower of London near a woman curled up with a novel on a comfy couch. And in the kitchen, the woman I loved, making coffee for herself and breakfast for the rest of us.

I'd only met her relatives a couple of times, but I loved them all. L. and I were on the verge of getting engaged, and they were going to be my family. I was so grateful to have so many good people in my life, people I really cared about.

My chief agenda that week was to help L. reconnect with her family. Among other things, this meant that I volunteered to make trips to the grocery store. In fact, by the end of our stay at that house, L. had no idea where the grocery store even was. And this was meaningful to me because it was such a departure for her from her previous life. Every time we needed something, someone would make a list and off I'd go. And no sooner than I got back L. would say, "We forgot so-and-so." And off I'd go again. And sometime in the pre-dinner hour someone would come up with a brilliant idea for what would make the perfect dessert, and off I'd go.

I happily made those trips, the car window rolled down, my hair blowing in the breeze, the music she loved playing on the stereo, glad that I could relieve the others of this task so they could continue to talk and read and swim in the fathoms-deep frigid water of the biggest lake this side of the Mississippi. And as they admired the sun-sparkled lake with the sound of loons traveling through the air, maybe some doors would open for them, too.

One day we all went on an afternoon picnic to a small lake nearby. Again, being with all of them, I felt that joyful buzz of activity. I watched L. go in the water, not far from shore, where she was joined by her mother. Before long they were swimming in the deeper waters, and then they were leisurely crossing the lake, and the next time I looked, they had reached the other shore and were stretched out, basking in the sun, on a rickety dock that led to an overgrown field of tall, summer-green grass. L. hadn't planned this adventure, and because the swim had spontaneously happened, she hadn't checked in with me, and what that meant was something a bit unusual: I was left to look after the boy.

I haven't talked much about the boy, have I? He was L.'s second child, the son who was born a year after her first son died. I was there when he entered the world (he was just a few minutes old when I met him), I babysat him (his was the only diaper I've changed in my life), and after L. and I got together, I sometimes picked him up from school or guitar lessons (he was the only child I had a conversation with by way of the rearview mirror), and now he was almost six. The three of us (L., the boy, and I) did many things together, and I remember one night in particular when we were upstairs in our new home after dinner. L. had been supervising the boy's bedtime routine, helping him change into his desired PJs, overseeing the brushing of his teeth, etc., and as usual, after doing the dishes, I found them in his bedroom, where she was propped up in his tiny bed next to him, reading from a book about a boy wizard who had once felt very alone in the world.

I sat on the floor beside the bed, leaned my back against the wall, and she handed me the book. She nestled down beside her child under the covers, and I picked up the epic tale where she'd left off. The boy was utterly enchanted by this story, a story we'd been reading for months, and as I read, L. closed her eyes and drifted into an exhausted half sleep that a mother like her has well earned. After a few more pages, and then a requested few more pages, and then okay-just-one-more additional page, it was time for the boy to go to sleep. I closed the book and went over to whisper good night to him. And the boy did something different. He reached up for a hug, and when I bent over, the boy wrapped his arms around my neck and kissed me—for the first time ever—and right then and there, he had me forever. I was a goner.

After that, the boy and I spent more time together, just the two of us. He was dead set against using the low children's basketball hoop, so I taught him how to throw the basketball so it could almost reach the rim of the adult one, and then I taught him how to get the basketball to touch the rim, and then I taught him how to get the basketball through the rim. On his mom's birthday, I took him to the beads-and-crafts store and he made some jewelry for her. I picked him up from school, put him in his car seat, and talked to him about his busy day while keeping an eye on him in the rearview mirror. I drove him to his guitar lessons where his little hands tried to operate the big guitar. And—because he had fallen in love with pinball when we visited Colorado the previous summer—I took him to an old downtown bar where I knew there was a great pinball machine, and he played as many quarters as he wanted, and we drank old-fashioned chocolate milkshakes straight from the metal cups they'd been blended in.

One Valentine's Day I wanted to do something special for him. He was already getting lots of candy and other great gifts that his great-gift-giving mother had thought of. So I went to a local gallery where I'd previously bought a couple of decorative birds for L. One of the birds was black and the other was blue and they were made out of sticks and had fake feathers and beaded eyes. But now the artist had made a red one, and as soon as I saw it, I knew it was the perfect gift for the boy. It was red, which was fitting for Valentine's Day, and this boy, though very much a child, also enjoyed the occasional foray into the adult world. (For instance, he had a growing collection of ties that, occasionally, when the whim struck, he liked to wear to school.)

Buckbee & Fitzgerald

So I wrapped up this bird in fancy wrapping paper and I gave it to him on February 14, that day set aside for love, and indeed he did like it, just as I thought he would. I explained to him that his new bird could fit in with the two other birds that L. had set up on top of the upright piano when we moved into our new house. "You can be the red bird," I told the boy. "Your mom and I can be the other two birds, and we can be a family together."

And so there we stood, in bird form, three birds in a little cluster, and every day when I strolled home from the university after teaching class and came through the front door and walked down the hall toward the voices in the kitchen that fucking cat—

(Sorry! My dictation took an odd turn there because those are the words I just uttered when I saw the orange cat, the same orange cat I saw yesterday, slipping through a gap in the fence into my yard and adopting a prowling-for-pigeons posture.)

One of the advantages of dictating—instead of writing—is I can be on the lookout for predators like this fucking cat while I "write." This time I didn't rush to the door and throw it open to scare the bejesus out of the cat like I did yesterday. Instead, I bided my time. I tiptoed to the door, I watched, I waited, and when the cat was well away from the fence, and totally lost in a sniffing reverie, I picked up a couple of mostly empty pop cans (my ammo), quietly turned the doorknob, and began to sprint toward him. The cat freaked. (Yes, I do feel bad for the cat . . . I love cats.) At first, he tried to get out the same way he had come into the yard, but he couldn't find the gap, and so he sprinted toward the gate, and I sprinted after him, jumping over the Stonehenge-like assembly of river rocks that I set up as a perimeter wall for the pigeons and ducking beneath the dangerously low limbs of the ancient plum trees until I cornered the cat by the gate and proceeded to launch the soda cans at it. The cans had just enough liquid in them to be able to travel a distance, but not enough to hurt the cat if I hit it. The cat, in the throes of the exact kind of panic I desired for him, finally scrambled up the chicken wire that covers the gate and disappeared around the corner. I haven't seen him in my yard since.

THE WOMAN I LOVED was on the dock with her mother on the far side of the lake, and the boy and I stood on the shore and looked at each other. His mother had left him without a word or any guidance, and she was way off on her own, and it was like we were both thinking, "Now what?"

Earlier, the boy's two cousins—who were also off on their own—had found a rope tied to a tree limb that extended over the lake. Maybe there was a small tire or slab of wood at the bottom of it, I can't remember for sure. What I do remember is standing at the edge of the lake with the boy, and he looked up at me and said, "I want to try."

He was genuinely scared, but it was also his nature to be curious and determined, and he waited for my answer.

The day before, we had driven into the national park that was not far from our rented vacation house. (We had so many people we had to take two separate cars!) I'm sure for people who grew up in big families, this buzz of activity is normal, but I was giddy from it. We saw the waterfalls and the goats and the glaciers that are on fast retreat, and at the pass I took a family picture with all of them in it, and then they insisted that a stranger take a picture so that I could be included, and then I was just another person in our group, looking like I belonged as much as anyone else.

In the early afternoon we pulled off the road and had a make-shift picnic. I was by the coolers, squatting down, retrieving something for somebody, when I noticed the boy was sitting on a pylon, about three feet off the ground, eating a sandwich, happy as could be. Just as I had the thought that he shouldn't be sitting

Buckbee & Fitzgerald

there, I saw him begin to tilt backwards. I jumped toward the boy, but there was no way I could close the gap in time, and I watched as he tumbled backwards and landed on the hard ground.

He was scared, of course, and he was crying, but we quickly saw that he was otherwise fine. His mother provided him with the comfort he needed, and in a few minutes the boy was back to eating a sandwich and smiling.

I felt something odd in that moment when the boy tumbled, like something had shifted inside me. Like a switch had been flipped. I knew that I had become the boy's shepherd. And I also knew that something such as this would never happen again, not while I was around, not on my watch. This new feeling, a singleness of focus, a determined protectiveness, is maybe something all parents have felt before. But it was new to me. And it was similar to the feeling I would have years later with Two-Step when he landed in the middle of the road and got hit by a car.

On the drive home, we passed a herd of elk drifting like ghosts across a field in the fading light, and as we silently watched them—L. by my side in the passenger seat, her mother and the boy in back—I was sure that I would never experience aloneness again.

———

SO AT THE LAKE, when the boy asked me if he could swing out over the water on the rope, I thought of all the things that could go wrong. He'd never done anything like this and he might not know when to let go and he might not know how to hold on and he might get his foot caught in the tire (or slat of wood or rope loop or whatever was at the bottom of the rope). But the athlete in me, this uber-Brian 1.0 part, this thing I had been nurturing since I was a little boy, in my backyard, with my mother at the kitchen sink looking out the window as I threw a baseball up in the air over and over and over again and dove across the lawn to make catch after catch in my grass-stained Wrangler jeans, knew that it was safe. I knew that if the boy let go too early, I could reach him in time, and I knew that the water was shallow enough that I could move at the same pace as the swinging rope, and I knew that if he somehow got tangled up in the rigging, he wouldn't be too high for me to reach him.

And so I said, "Yes, you can do this if you want." He sure looked nervous, but he also looked—and this part is hard to explain—like he now knew something about me, too. I could see it in him, in the way he looked at me, and that is that I could be trusted, even during what must have felt like a terrifying feat, and that he would be safe. So this determined boy, with his sweaty blond hair stuck to his forehead, stepped into the shallow water. I crouched down and took hold of him beneath his arms, the bare skin of my hands on his bare skin, and because I was an athlete, and I had energy and capacity, I did something that I would be unable to do now. I hoisted him up, and he grabbed onto the rope, and I pulled it back toward land so that he could swing . . . and I let go.

The rope was swinging, the boy was swinging, and I dashed into the water, and the boy let go just when he was supposed to, and he dropped into the water and into my waiting hands. I let him slip beneath the surface and pulled him back up and he looked happy and relieved, the way a child who is doing something beyond his years should look. And then he asked, "Can I do it again?" And I said, "Of course."

I'm sure the boy wished his mother could have witnessed his daring feat, but she was barely visible on the other side of the lake, stretched out in her bikini in the warming sun next to her mother, from whom she had been distanced of late. For the moment it was just him and me, together, in our own little bubble of togetherness.

Buckbee & Fitzgerald

I still dream about the boy all the time. When I wake up in the morning, I'm so glad I got to see him. In the dreams he is always the same age he was when he so bravely, so happily swung off that rope with me waiting beneath to catch him. He is always almost six.

———

NOT TOO MANY YEARS LATER, a number of my belongings that had been in the house I shared with L. and the boy showed up on the porch of the house I'm in now. Along with a pile of clothes and books and random pieces of domestic detritus was a box containing the red bird that I'd given to the boy. I will never know if the boy ever found out that his bird was even missing.

———

MY EDITOR'S NAME IS CAROL ANN. Whenever I have a written-in-my-head, dictated-while-suffering-a-terrific-headache, and semi-polished-by-trying-to-edit-the-words-on-a-screen chunk of story, I send it off to her. She is a wind-in-the-sails kind of person, kind in her words, not shy with praise or encouragement, and, honestly, it helps keep me going. This, I realize, is kind of a strange moment in the dictation for her, because she will soon be reading what I just said about her, and this must present some sort of dilemma, because she has to choose whether to edit herself out, or keep herself in, or maybe change the way I described her. But I don't mind putting this onus on her because, to be honest, I'm a little mad at her.

I talked to her yesterday about the lake house and the boy. She said, "It kind of feels like you're idealizing L." And I said, "Well, yeah." Then she said, "I think the reader is going to want to learn a little bit more about the complexity of the relationship." And then I had to say something that was not very nice to my editor. I said, "I'm sorry, but in this case, I can't help the reader." What I meant but didn't say was that my memory of L. was sacred, and I didn't want to make it even the slightest bit profane.

———

I WAS SITTING in the morning sun outside a coffee shop while talking on the phone with my editor. She is pulling oceans of story out of me so that she will know which little wave should come next.

The weather this fall in western Montana has been incredible. It's the kind of season people a hundred years from now will talk about. There was the winter of '96, and now the fall of '22. The coffee shop's resident cat knew how great the weather was. While I talked with my editor about the reader's looming disappointment, the cat lay on its side next to me, soaking up the sun, sometimes pressing her curled paws against the backrest of the bench as if she were kneading dough. Behind the coffee shop is an irrigation channel, an offshoot of the Clark Fork River. The channel is wide and shallow at some points, and narrow and deep at others. This little stream of water happens to be the same stream that Two-Step landed next to, about half a mile downstream from the coffee shop, when he got hit by the car. That day was a mirror of yesterday, the spring equivalent to a perfect fall day, the temperature a little cool, the sun warm, the grass and bushes and trees startling everyone with their bright colors.

I saw Two-Step—

Sorry, I had to stop the dictation right there. A friend of mine just called. She said she was downtown and had come out of the gym and saw a pigeon fall off the flat roof and injure itself, and now it couldn't fly and could I help. I really have no room to take in any more injured birds, and the bigger issue is I really have no more physical capacity to help them, but I said yes.

I wanted to help the pigeon, but I also wanted to help my friend, because she is a lover of vulnerable creatures, and she was very upset. I tried to give her advice over the phone, but I could tell she was distraught and unsure what to do, so I said, "Wait where you are and make sure nobody runs over the bird and I'll be right there." When I arrived, she was in tears, and an adult pigeon lay in the street, and to me it was clear that it was mortally wounded. But I told my friend I could help the pigeon. I told her at the very least I could give it a dark, quiet, comfortable place to rest in the spare room in my house. And so he is in a box lined with a soft pillow sham right now. This is the same room where Two-Step lived for a short while when he first came into my life, and the same room where I put Popcorn when he was sick and where he died. It is dark and warm and quiet in there; probably the only thing the pigeon can hear is the muffled sound of my dictating voice through the closed door.

I just got off the couch and turned the furnace on for the first time this year. Winter is coming. I just checked on the injured pigeon, and he is dead.

I'VE BROKEN all my own rules. I was never going to use social media. After that went out the window, I told myself I wouldn't post more than two or three times on Facebook. Then when that plan didn't work out, I swore that no matter what, I would never tell a sad animal story. Clearly, I've tossed that one aside, too.

There was a time in my life after my mother got sick when I simply couldn't bear to hear any more sad animal stories, no matter how small. If you are close to the edge of a cliff, a story like that can give you an unexpected push.

Once, after I got home from work, the person I was living with at the time started to tell me about something that had happened that day, and it involved a bat in a perilous situation. I wouldn't let her speak. I think I rudely cut her off. I didn't want to hear about one of those furry, big-eyed, bighearted creatures we're disappearing from the planet. Now, of course, I feel bad for forcing her to be alone with her sad story.

I guess I'm susceptible to troubling thoughts right now, because the loss of this injured pigeon has catapulted me right into them. The only thing that matters is that all the other birds are in the house tonight. I'm going to make sure the doors are locked and the alarm is set and the trip wire is connected to the dynamite.

———

WHEN TWO-STEP got hit by the car, he soared way up in the sky—I saw a few feathers floating in the air—and then he fell to earth in some bushes on the other side of the road. I sprinted toward him, cursing at the retreating Subaru, and looked for him in the tightly packed bushes, the ones that bordered the irrigation channel I was just talking about. I thought it would take a miracle for Two-Step to have survived, and I figured it would be a miracle if I could even find him. But I was lucky that day, and maybe the God that I met in my ketamine dream was with me, because it took me about thirty seconds. He was on the ground, standing between two bushes, mostly hidden in the shadows beneath the low tangle of branches. He was quivering, I suppose because he was in shock. Or maybe he was scared, and he was quivering the way pigeons do when they see a hawk or smell a stupid cat. I got down on my knees and talked softly to him. "It's okay, it's okay." I guess you could say I cooed to him, but it was hard to speak the words because my heart was in my throat.

I slowly reached my hands toward Two-Step, and his quivering increased and he tried to move deeper into the bushes. I knew I only had one chance to grab him, and so I reached out as fast as I could, but it wasn't fast enough. He squirmed out of my fingers and got on the other side of the bushes, inches away from the edge of the slope that dropped down into the irrigation channel.

I sprang to my feet and ran along the bushes, looking for a gap to slip through. I couldn't find one, so I raised my arms to cover my face and used my body to break through. I saw Two-Step maybe fifteen feet upstream, and he was walking in little circles, oblivious to where he was, and then he took one step too close to the edge and he tumbled down the slope and into the rushing water.

I got on my butt and slid down the slope into the channel. The water was deeper there, thigh-high and moving fast. My shoes got stuck in the muck and it felt like I was moving through quicksand. Two-Step was thrashing in the water, spinning in circles while flapping his wings furiously to keep them above the waterline. I finally made it to the middle of the channel and got myself ready to catch him.

Behind me was a big irrigation pipe, and I knew if Two-Step got past me, he would be swept into the pipe and taken underground. Mind you, this was all unfolding very fast, and before I knew it, he was right in front of me, and I had my one chance, and I didn't miss. I scooped him up and pulled him close to my chest, just like L. did when she saved the baby goose. He was still fighting me, but I wasn't going to let him go, no matter what.

There we were, man and bird, frozen in time. I stood very still, and I could feel his breathing, his expanding chest against my chest. And I suppose he felt my breathing, too, my expanding chest against his. And then he calmed down. I rearranged my grip so I could hold his wings firmly against his body. Pigeons generally don't like to be held this way, but I have learned that if they find purchase with their feet, so they aren't dangling in the air, they are okay with it. Without unwrapping my other fingers, I loosened my pinkies, and I felt Two-Step's feet moving around, seeking a landing spot, until he found them, and I felt his soft feet, one gripping my left pinkie, one gripping my right.

All I had to figure out was how to get out of the muck, climb up the slick slope, and pass through the thick, dense bushes, all while holding Two-Step firmly in my two hands. I managed not to slip on the slope, and I made it up to the edge, and I turned away from the bushes and hunched over so that my body was protecting Two-Step, and then I backed through them. I got scraped but it didn't matter, because Two-Step was fine, at least for the moment. I figured what would happen to him in the coming hours was the same thing that happened to most of the birds that my mother and I tried to save when I was a child. An injured bird would look okay, then you'd put him in a box and when you went to check on him later, he would be dead.

I got Two-Step home and my migraine exploded, but the pain this time didn't incapacitate me. I placed Two-Step in a shallow box that I'd lined with soft fabric and put the box on my kitchen table. I retreated to my spot on the couch, and that's how we spent the day. I would lean forward, holding my head in my hands, and every now and again look up to check on Two-Step. And he would be in his box, not having moved at all, and he'd be looking back at me.

Later, I looked up and saw that he was standing up in the box, and then he flew to the top of the refrigerator. I couldn't believe what I was seeing—my pigeon rising from the ashes.

I brought Two-Step his cup of water and I broke up some peanuts into smaller pieces and scattered them on top of the refrigerator. And not much later he had a drink, and not much later he began walking around on top of the refrigerator, pecking

Buckbee & Fitzgerald

at the peanuts. He'd just been hit by a Subaru and now he was having dinner.

Still, I was scared when I went to bed that night. I tried not to think about what I might wake up to. One of the upsides of this constant pain is that it exhausts me so much that, unlike in my earlier life when I had bad bouts of insomnia, I fall asleep right away. I'm sure I dreamed, but I can't remember now what about, and the next thing I was aware of was a familiar clicking sound outside my closed bedroom door. It was the sound of Two-Step's feet against the hardwood floor, and he was pacing, as usual, wanting me to get out of bed. (Maybe he wanted to be sure I was okay.) So I got out of bed and walked to the door and opened it, and there was my friend.

———

I HAVE BEEN PROMISING my editor for some time that I would write about the dreadful thing that happened last May. I have been putting it off, to say the least.

She has been gently hounding me to fill in this missing part of the book, and I've promised her repeatedly that I will get to it. It is obvious that I have some issues related to this event, and recently she has started telling me that maybe I don't really need to write about it at all. She is worried about my pain.

But this far into the story I don't feel like I have a choice.

It happened right after Mother's Day, on the day I got the first of my multiple COVID boosters. (These shots are recommended for people with ME/CFS.) I kept the front door closed that morning so my flock of unsupervised birds would be forced to stay inside until I got home from the pharmacy. After I returned, having somehow managed to avoid unleashing a monster headache while driving through the bright sunshine, I opened the door and all the birds flew out, including the one with mostly black feet,

Two-Step's baby, who I was telling you about earlier. I knew that unlike the other birds, who would be outside until evening, my little buddy would only stay outside for a short time, and then he would flap his way inside and return to his perch on the windowsill, from where he would watch me watching him. I think it made us both feel calm to gaze at one another like this.

I slowly ate a very light lunch, knowing I would soon feel sick from the shot I'd just received. I was eagerly anticipating that feeling, because, as I have learned, the flu-like symptoms that come with vaccines seem to push aside my other pains—the three-and-a-half-year-old headache (a toddler now) and the post-exertional body aches—giving me what feels like a pleasant break from those familiar afflictions.

It may sound strange to be excited about feeling sick, but having low-grade flu symptoms always reminds me of my mother taking care of me when I was ill as a child, bringing me a cup of sherbet and pressing the back of her hand against my warm forehead. And the dreams that accompany the great deep sleep of a mild sickness! I would live in those dreams if I could.

I have also learned that—for whatever reason—the naps I take when I get vaccine-sick never result in even a hint of migraine. And so on that day, I knew I would be able to take my first nap in a long time (ever since my first COVID shot) and maybe spend quality time in that other world with the woman I loved and the boy I missed.

Every few minutes, as I sat on my well-worn spot on the couch, I would glance out the window to check on the birds. Many of them had gathered around the lilac bush, but I also had a good view of the rest of the yard, and I felt at ease that all my birds were safe.

My little buddy, the young pigeon who had been born in the house over the winter, was in the dappled shade under the lilac bush, his wings twitching and his throat pulsing, which is what birds do when they are beginning to experience the big, beautiful world that awaits them and they are nervously excited or excitedly nervous.

I returned to my lunch, expecting him to join me in the house shortly.

A few minutes later, when I looked out the window again, I saw the birds beneath the lilac bush, but this time there was a visitor I hadn't seen before, and it was a hawk.

The hawk—a midsize hawk, not as big as a red-tailed hawk, but not as small as a sharp-shinned hawk—was standing on top of a pigeon.

I jumped up and began cursing and ran the four or five strides to my front door. When I stepped off the porch, the hawk was maybe ten feet from me, but despite my sudden, noisy appearance, he didn't fly away. He stayed where he was, on top of the pigeon. So I ran at him, and finally he took off. But he only flew to the low branches of the neighbor's giant pine, where he settled and literally hawk-eyed the spot he had just left. Without taking my eyes off him, I bent down and gathered some small stones from my neglected garden, stones hefty enough to travel a distance, but light enough not to do any real harm if they hit their mark.

In all my years as an athlete, I doubt I ever performed anything more skillfully than I did that day. Maybe it was thanks to all the balls I tossed in the air as a child, showing off for my mother. The first stone I threw threaded through the pine-needled branches and passed the hawk by no more than two inches. I was probably thirty feet away. (In fact, it was forty feet; I just measured it.) The hawk was startled by that first projectile, but he didn't move, so I threw a second stone, and this one somehow came even closer to him than the first one, and it scared him, and he unclenched his talons from the branch and flew off.

I wasn't rid of him, however, because he only flew a few yards, landing on the low, slightly slanted roof of my neighbor's house.

I should interject here that I love hawks. The first person who helped me save Two-Step's life was herself a raptor rehabilitator. (I donate money to her from time to time and am now the proud sponsor of an owl named Merlin.) I also know it is possible that the hawk was sticking around because it had hungry eyases, or baby hawks, to feed. It makes me sad to think of those little guys missing a very necessary meal because of me. But what about my birds?

The hawk was staring intently at the ground beneath the lilac bush, so I threw another stone that came even closer to him. He retreated to a higher, more distant part of the neighbor's roof. So I took the biggest stone I had—one that I knew could hurt if it hit him—and I threw it.

I had calculated that if I skimmed the stone along the roof, like a rock on a river, its momentum would be slowed enough to not cause any significant harm if it struck the hawk. Maybe my mother from above was in control of my aim that day, because the stone did exactly what I hoped, and it grazed the hawk, and this time he took off for real.

What came next was the hard part. The bird that the hawk had attacked hadn't moved and was still under the lilac bush. I knew it wasn't Two-Step or V., but it could have been anybody else.

Even before I got close, I could tell the bird was dead. I knelt beside him, and I nudged him gently so I could get a look at his legs and feet. I didn't want harm to come to any pigeon, but I prayed the legs and feet of this dead bird were pink or red. But his legs and feet were black. I realized then that it was my little friend, my windowsill companion.

I felt overwhelmed with dark thoughts, like the ones I had when I hit the bird in the Great Basin and realized that the world is shitty and so is mankind and so am I. But this was even worse.

At that moment I knew that I had to get him buried—and fast—because a tidal wave of grief was coming. I knew precisely where I would bury him (beneath the pedestal birdbath, where I had buried other birds), and I knew what I would use as a marker, and it would be the only one in the yard (a jagged slat of wood left over from building the nesting box), and I knew what I would wrap around his still-very-warm body (a piece of the floral cloth that I had used as an awning for Two-Step's first outdoor hutch).

That fabric was getting smaller and smaller, and I often wondered what would run out first—the cloth, the pigeons, or me. I tried not to think about that as I rushed to the task at hand. But on my way to retrieve the cloth from the shed, I hesitated and changed course, retreating instead to my living room, where I took watch at the window.

The hawk had been so reluctant to leave the bird he had killed that I suspected he was going to return to claim his kill. I wanted to teach him a lesson, dammit, and scare him so good that he'd never come back. And, I am ashamed to admit, I also wanted him to return so that I could make *him* feel afraid, feel terror, feel small and helpless.

I had collected an assortment of lightweight balls—old tennis balls and racquetballs—so that I could throw them at any stupid cat that dared breach the perimeter of my yard, and I grabbed a few of them and stood at that window, waiting.

Within two minutes, the hawk returned. He swept right down to the body of my dead friend and resumed his position. As he swiveled his head, he looked fierce and—I suppose—beautiful.

This time I didn't rush out of the house. I tiptoed through the open door and off the porch, and, with fifteen feet of yard separating us, we stared at each other. The racquetball was the first ball I threw—it was the lightest of the three—and it bounced off the ground next to the hawk and startled him.

He immediately spread his wings to fly away, which was exactly what I hoped he would do. But he also did something I hadn't foreseen. Despite being a smallish hawk, he managed to lift off with my dead friend gripped in his talons.

I instantly became aware of my predicament. If the hawk flew beyond the perimeter of my yard, he would be gone for good, and this was unacceptable to me, because at that moment nothing mattered as much as placing my pigeon in the ground, where he would be next to the other birds. I wanted to always know where he was.

The hawk flew around the lilac bush and beneath the low limbs of a tall plum tree, and I hurled the first tennis ball at him. Again, I came within a few inches of hitting him, so close that he responded by trying to ascend higher. He was struggling, though, from the weight of my dead friend, and his wings were flapping furiously.

Do you know those movies where an airplane tries to gain altitude at the last possible second to avoid slamming into a mountain? That's the image that popped into my head. The hawk was going to get to the border of my yard, point his beak skyward, and attempt to eclipse the tall branches of the short plum trees, his cargo in tow, and from there it would be a smooth escape.

I had only one more chance to stop him, and I drew my arm back and launched the second tennis ball. He was farther away now, forty feet or more, but fortunately my aim was true, and as the ball whizzed past him, he dropped the little pigeon, and then he shot upward, and he cleared a thicket of twisted trees with dead branches, and he was gone.

I picked up my friend and cupped his soft warmth in my hands. I dashed to the house for the scissors, dashed to the shed for the cloth, dashed to the corner of the neglected garden for the shovel, and then I went to the graveyard I'd made, and I put him in the ground.

It so happens that I am being interrupted at this very moment by a bird of prey, even as I dictate the last part of this dreadful thing. I am sitting in the shade of my yard in a pocket of air cooled by the nearby Clark Fork River. Not too high in the sky is an osprey (sometimes misidentified as a sea hawk). He is soaring in small circles, occasionally pausing in midair as if contemplating a dive. He hasn't done so yet. I know exactly where his nest is, even though I can't walk that far anymore. Ospreys return to the same nest every year, and they live a long time, twenty years or more. In previous years, when I could easily walk to his nest (and well beyond it), I would hear his chicks squeaking with urgent delight when he or his partner returned with a trout. I don't have the same kind of ambivalence for the osprey that I do for the hawk or the owl, because ospreys don't attack pigeons. And somehow, mysteriously, the pigeons know that. They don't even blink when an osprey strays a little far afield over my house. The osprey might as well be a sparrow or a chickadee or even a crow (which, despite its size, doesn't alarm the pigeons one bit).

I remember the first time a hawk came to my yard. Two-Step alerted me to its arrival by displaying behavior I had never seen before. We were in the house, and he was on top of the refrigerator, and suddenly he flew across the kitchen, landing on the counter beneath an overhanging cabinet, and proceeded to make short grunting noises, a sound I'd never heard from him before. I didn't know what was wrong, but when I looked out the screen door, I saw a hawk on a nearby branch of the boxelder maple, and he was facing in the direction of my house.

The thing is, I have no idea how Two-Step knew the hawk was there. From his place on the refrigerator, he couldn't see the hawk. Did he hear the whisper of the hawk's feet as they landed on the branch? Did he smell its predatory scent? Or could he sense the great shadow that only a hawk can cast? It's a mystery. Another wonderful, beautiful mystery that I guess has something to do with what pigeons have learned in the millions of years they've spent on earth while facing threats from all directions.

There is no action in the sky above me. The osprey has moved on, and now so will I.

After burying my friend, I collapsed on the rumpled covers of my unmade bed and fell into a deep sleep. A couple of hours later, when I woke up, I felt bad for falling asleep so quickly. But I have learned from experience that grief—for me, at least—is the best sleeping aid in the world.

I feel stupid. I delayed and delayed in telling this part of the story, and now I have gone on and on about it. The simple truth is that this dreadful thing was tragic (to me), but it's the kind of ordinary event that happens all the time in the lives of birds.

Now, when I sit on my couch every day and look out the window, I can't help but think of that young bird perched on the windowsill. Sometimes I can hear the soft sounds Two-Step and V. make when they're cuddling together in the nesting box mounted on the outside of the window. And the feeling I get is both peaceful and terrible.

I lost a friend that day. I guess it is that simple. And as a result, I have been more alone since he left.

There is one more thing. It still hurts to think about it.

The part I left out is that when I went to my friend, the fallen pigeon, I saw that the hawk had not yet pulled a single feather from him, which means the attack had just happened. If I had looked out the window just twenty seconds earlier, or even just ten, I might have been able to save my friend. Why didn't I look sooner? Was I too focused on eating my lunch? Was I too busy watching some stupid TV show? Why can't I unwind time and just look a few seconds sooner?

When I first found my pigeon friend, after scaring the hawk away, and I saw his familiar black legs and black toes, I noticed something else. The bird was completely intact, but his head was missing.

I searched the yard, but I didn't find the rest of him. I gathered up his body and held it in my hands, the same way I held him when he was a baby. I felt his weight, his considerable weight, his warm should-be-alive weight, and then I placed him in the earth.

I have many birds buried in different parts of my yard, but this is the only grave that is marked.

———

THE IDEA OF MONTANA first got planted in my head when I was still in high school. Montana represented remoteness, natural beauty, and adventure. In Montana, I wouldn't be surrounded by lawyers and bankers, and I wouldn't feel the pressure to be a lawyer or banker, and I wouldn't feel ashamed for not being a lawyer or banker. I could easily imagine myself alone there without feeling alone. This was back in 1985, mind you, when such places still existed in the Lower 48.

I finally saw Montana for the first time when I drove from Chicago to look for a place to rent while I attended grad school in Missoula in 1997. It was midsummer, and everything was so clear—the air, the sky, the water. Every time I drove past a hillside, I felt the inclination to pull the car over and run up it.

I soon learned some of Montana's quirks. For instance, when I moved to Montana there was no daytime speed limit on the highways. The only time Montana had a speed limit was during the energy crisis in the '70s, when the federal government mandated it. But even then, Montana dodged it almost entirely. Sure, they posted the occasional speed limit sign, which drivers would rarely follow, and yes, the police occasionally wrote tickets. But if you did get pulled over, the citation wasn't for "speeding," it was for "wasting fuel." All tickets, no matter how fast you were driving (unless you were reckless), were five bucks.

One of the first things that thrilled me in Missoula was seeing a CATTLE AT LARGE sign. Until that moment, "at large" suggested only criminals and escaped convicts to me. That sign made me think about cows differently. Were they really just innocently chewing grass on the side of the road? Or were they ruminating on dark thoughts and schemes? What was behind those big black eyes? I remember one time when I was driving on a remote back road at fifty miles an hour, I saw a CATTLE AT LARGE sign as I came around a bend. That sign instructed me to slow down, which was a good thing because there was suddenly a big shadow ahead of me, a shadow I might have driven right through if I hadn't seen that sign, a shadow that was actually a very large cow lying halfway across my lane.

The expression "at large" means "with great liberty," or, essentially, having a large amount of space to roam. It's exactly what the young characters in Bruce Springsteen's songs are looking for—to be at large. Montana has those signs because this is a state with places where there are lots of cows but no fences, places where you'll be driving a hundred miles and suddenly encounter a herd of thousand-pound animals milling around in the road in no particular hurry to get out of your way. It is not that different from what is going on in my house at this very moment, a house that is filled with many pigeons at large, a house where there is no divide between "our" world and the natural world. I may have left the metropolis behind long ago, but it seems I'm now situated neatly in what I've come to call Pigeonopolis.

ONE OF THE YOUNG PIGEONS is spraddle-legged. Even when he was a baby, I could tell that he had a difficult time keeping his legs under him. His left leg dragged behind him, causing the hip joint to turn backwards. At first, I tried to tie his legs together, but that didn't work. I finally resorted to buying tags, plastic cuffs that clip on to the bird's leg just below the knee. I doubled up some yarn and knotted it to each cuff, so that his feet couldn't move too far apart and the soft yarn wouldn't chafe his belly too bad.

I left the cuffs on for a few weeks, until he was a young juvenile, and then I removed them, and he was able to keep both his feet mostly under him. But within a few days the bad leg had spraddled again, and the hip joint was turned in the wrong direction. He is disabled, but he tries so hard to be a "normal" bird that he has become one of my favorites. He's on the floor of my living room, right in the middle of the wide doorway to the kitchen, and he's looking at me. Every time I walk past him, he gets scared, but it is still his favorite place in the house and he won't budge from it.

In the cabinet on the hearth is the juvenile pigeon the neighbors brought to me, the one with the broken wing. And there is one other juvenile in my living room, the beautiful bastard child of my caged female and the male "bully" pigeon who nests in a box on the porch that I installed for Two-Step and V. last year (but which they never took to). I know who the juvenile's father is because he doesn't resemble his mom or her partner in the slightest, but he looks identical to the bully pigeon. I guess there must have been a day a few months ago when I rolled the cage out onto the porch, opened the cage door so the flightless couple could stroll around the yard for a bit, and in that time, she had a quick—and consequential—affair with him. But the thing is, her partner still totally loves her. They do everything together. When I let them out, they waddle to the far end of the lawn side by side, and if he is pecking at dandelion leaves, she's pecking at dandelion leaves. In the cage, they stand pressed closely together, wing to wing.

Anyway, that beautiful bastard is walking around my living room, very much at large, looking for a place on the floor to nestle into.

This bird activity is a good distraction for me. It is also quite meditative and seems to soothe my headache. At certain times of the day all three of these young pigeons begin preening their feathers, making a rhythmic flicking sound that fills the room.

Two-Step and V. are in their nesting box beside me, on the other side of the window, where they get some of the warmth that radiates from the house. I just twisted the rod to close the blinds and so now maybe it feels more like night in there, and they can practice regular bird hours and go to sleep. Soon I will go to sleep, too, and in our dreams, we will all be safe.

I DIDN'T DO as my editor asked. I didn't talk about the complicated parts of the relationship I had with L. But here's the thing: I was friends with L. for several years, and then we were together for several years, and in that time, there weren't a lot of conflicts to talk about (other than the ones we faced together, like how our friends did not approve of us being together, which seemed to be especially challenging for L.).

L. and I had some minor arguments, like everyone does, and we made up, and we weren't always at our best, but we showed up for each other when needed or not, and we were kind and caring. Things hadn't always been easy for her, and then she suffered the hardest loss a parent can suffer. You don't need the specifics about the time we bickered about this or that, do you? You've been in relationships, you know how they go. And if you have been in a good relationship, a really good one, then you know how wonderful that feels. Things were good, for a long time, and then quite suddenly they weren't.

Part 4

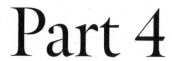

(OCTOBER–DECEMBER 2022)

THE FIRST ANIMAL THAT I KNEW WELL WHO DIED WAS Max. Max was my friend, the family dog we got when I was four. He was the Two-Step of dogs.

I can't remember what famous writer explored the paradox of how everyone thinks they are really funny, but hardly anyone actually is. The same is true with pet dogs: everyone thinks theirs is the most special, but they can't all be the most special. Max, however—and this was a verdict that came from people outside our family who knew him a little or a lot—was the most special dog.

In 1972, our family visited the animal shelter in Ossining, New York. I remember being there for what seemed like a long time as we looked at all the caged canines. We finally settled on a young German shepherd who seemed calm and friendly. We brought him home and my family was now complete—Mom, Dad, brother, dog. But that night we began talking about the dog we *didn't* bring home. The one that charged at the front of his enclosure when we came by, who made excited whimpering sounds as if talking to us. The dog we had brought home, the German shepherd, was behaving perfectly well, but somehow that other dog had gotten stuck in our heads.

So the next day we did something that I can't believe we did. We took the German shepherd *back* to the shelter and brought home Max, the excitable, shaggy, black-and-brown dog who had been hurling himself at us.

All these years later, I admit I'm still worried about what happened to that German shepherd. I hope he found a good home. He was a friendly dog, a good dog, and so I like to think someone with a big heart and an even bigger yard adopted him soon after we abandoned him. I get sad, thinking about the life he could have lived if he had stayed with us. Because we proved to be good dog owners, my mother in particular.

For instance, my mother—despite pretty much being the sole parent of two young boys—signed Max up for a weekly obedience course where she learned how to teach him to do things like sit and come and stay and heel. The effectiveness of his training became evident a couple of years later, when we moved to our house in the suburbs of Chicago. When we arrived, my mother put Max on his leash and walked him slowly around the edge of our half-acre lot. Then she walked him around again. And then she let Max off the leash, and for the next fifteen years he never left our property on his own.

When I walked home from school, or from the bus stop at the end of the road, Max was often sitting at the very corner of the yard waiting for me, wagging his tail, maybe letting out one of those excited whimpers of his. But he wouldn't take a step onto the street, and he wouldn't take a step onto the neighbor's property. He just waited. I don't know how long he waited—for hours sometimes, my mother said.

When Max was still a puppy, my mother was brushing him and found a brown bug on him. It was a tick. And my mother brushed a little more and found a few more ticks. She was concerned—there were so many ticks—and so she called the vet. The vet told my mom, "You can't kill ticks by squishing them with your fingers." And my mom asked how to kill them, and the vet said, "Do you have a wine bottle in the house?" She did, yes, and she proceeded to follow the vet's instructions. She put Max in the porcelain bathtub and applied some kind of powder or spray (or maybe it was just water), and the ticks began to fall off. One tick, two ticks, three ticks, four. My mom peeled the label off the wine bottle, leaned over the edge of the tub, and proceeded to roll the bottle over the tub's flat bottom. And when Max got out of the tub and the ticks kept falling off him, she rolled the bottle across the bathroom's tile floor. Her weight on the bottle was just enough pressure to squish the bugs. It was a massacre.

I wish my mother was around to tell me that story again, so I could get all of it right. And then I could ask her if she felt bad for the ticks. She was such a kindhearted, creature-loving woman, I'm sure she'd say yes.

———

MAX LIKED TO PLAY FETCH, and sometimes my brother and I would throw the ball and hide, and Max would come find us. When my brother and I played catch in the backyard, Max would run back and forth between us, waiting for an errant throw. But when the ball landed in a neighbor's yard, Max would charge all the way up to the invisible boundary—the one he had learned from my mom the one time she walked him around the yard—and stop.

When we moved to Chicago from New York, we had to put Max in a crate at the airport and check him with the baggage. Max was okay being put in the crate, but he did not at all like being separated from his family. Max only bit one person in his entire life and it was on that day, when he was not himself. I suppose he must have been abandoned once already, when he was a young puppy, and maybe he was afraid it was happening again. So he bit the baggage handler. I take some solace in thinking dogs probably bite those handlers all the time.

Before our plane took off that day, my father, who had worked as a detective for the biggest security company in the world and knew how to pull strings, arranged to visit Max outside the plane before he was loaded inside. I know my father didn't want to put our dog through any suffering, but I wonder what it felt like to him. I know what it would have felt like to my mother, but when

I think about what was going on in my father's heart, I am at a loss. He loved Max, but did he feel an agonizing pang as Max was loaded into the cargo hold of an airplane?

The best (and worst) of times with Max were when we went on one of our few family vacations. Max had to stay home, and it was really hard to say goodbye. But when we got back, we'd stand outside the side door and debate who would get the privilege of opening the door. I got to do it once or twice. When the door opened, Max would come running and I'd be the first person he saw. And he'd jump up on me (the only time he was allowed to do that) and he whimpered with such desperation you couldn't help but realize how much you loved him and how much he loved you, too. You don't feel alone when you have a dog like that.

———

UNLIKE LATER ON, my early childhood was pretty good. I had my dog, and my mom and I saved birds and she watched me catch balls in the yard, and I was good in school and liked by my classmates and my teachers. The question is: What happened to me after that? I remember one summer—maybe I was twelve— when I was so embarrassed by my thin legs that I didn't wear shorts the whole season. And I remember my father joking at the kitchen table, "Brian's so skinny he has to move around in the shower just to get wet." I don't think he was trying to hurt my feelings—that would come later. I think he was trying to minimize the issue, but of course it had the opposite effect. At thirteen I began to feel weak, by fifteen I felt freakishly so, and for the next few years I was terrified of being found out, that people would learn the secret of just how weak and pathetic I was.

———

Buckbee & Fitzgerald

Though I became more bitter and sulky the further I crept into adolescence, it didn't ever affect my feelings for Max. I was free to be a child with him, free to play, free of examination and judgment, confident of being loved. (I realize I just described exactly what it felt like to be with L.) I built snow forts for Max and taught him how to catch the Frisbee and he even seemed to welcome me dressing him up as Bruce Springsteen. Max was never allowed on the beds or furniture, but in my later high school years I would sit up in bed and pat the top of the covers, excitedly repeating, "Come on, come on, come on!" Max would anxiously pace back and forth at the foot of the bed, thinking something like, "Is this really happening? But isn't this wrong? I'm not supposed to be up there, right?" And then he'd decide, "What the hell." He was my first spooning partner.

MY THERAPIST FOLLOWS the classic psychoanalytic model, meaning she doesn't talk much and she almost never gives advice and she waits for me to make my own discoveries (which, as you can tell by now, doesn't happen very often). But yesterday she did something out of character. She decided to drive home a point, or maybe she wanted to say something she has been hold-ing in for the last seven years. "Those two words are different from all the others you use," she said. I didn't know what she was talking about. "What words?"

"'Weak,'" she said. "And 'pathetic.'"

She's right, though I don't like to confront my long history with these words. I was so afraid of being both those things that they have stuck with me through many decades and time zones. I have always been terrified of being found out. It's why in high school, when I ran track, I'd get sick before every race. It's why on spring break in Key West when I was twenty, I never wore a bathing suit. I didn't even wear shorts. I wore camo pants and a long-sleeve green-and-yellow rugby shirt the entire time.

One afternoon during that trip I was in the hotel room of two girls I was friends with, one of whom I thought could be "the one." I was so unthreatening to them that they were fine with all of us being in one bed together, under the covers. "You know," the girl I secretly loved said, "of all the guys in that giant group you came down here with, we like hanging out with you best." They'd clearly been having a conversation about me at an earlier time. What they said was a shock to me, because I *was* different from all the other guys. Those other guys were the ones girls liked (weren't they?). Those other guys weren't weak and pathetic.

I didn't try to kiss either of those girls at the time, and I certainly didn't confess my feelings. I just enjoyed the comfort, the coziness, the company. But I was still sure, if they saw me, if they *really* saw me, my secret would be revealed, and they'd find out the truth about me, and then I wouldn't be their favorite anymore.

Later that same year, my father pulled me out of college because my grades were so bad. Then I got booted from the house, too, and moved into the city and got a job working room service at a fancy hotel. One night I got a call from my parents and they told me I needed to come home. "It's time," my mother said. "Time for what?" I asked. "We're putting Max to sleep," she said. This quickly turned into another occasion where I could barely speak. "I'm not coming," I finally said. "I can't." They kept telling me I needed to be there and I kept telling them I couldn't. I felt weak and pathetic, but I didn't care one bit. Finally, my father said, "If you don't do this, you will regret it for the rest of your life."

Max was lying down in the kitchen on his side when the vet gave him the shot. My mother was kneeling next to him, leaning forward, her hand touching his head, and my father and brother were standing at what I guess felt like a safe distance, and I picked a spot behind all of them so no one would see me when I started crying.

———

I MENTIONED MY EDITOR TODAY to my pain reprocessing therapist. "A collaboration with a friend" was on the list of "things that I can do in my reduced state to reduce my pain." My pain reprocessing therapist smiled, genuinely glad I was in a collaboration, but then about ten minutes later she dumped me.

———

IT'S HARD TO SAY WHEN the door-opening really began. I don't think there was a specific moment; rather it was gradual and shaped by the confluence of a number of events—getting older, experiencing loss, feeling lost. When you are a child, there is no separation between you and the big world of wonder and mystery. There are no doors that need to be opened.

Maybe you are finally old enough to be outside in the middle of summer when something magical happens—it gets dark, very dark. Maybe at this moment you feel like you are getting away with something, and maybe you are, maybe your parents have had a drink too many and are letting things slide, maybe they are inside flirting with the neighbors who just dropped by, and if you can stay out of their sight, you can experience night—*really* experience it—for the first time.

My suburban backyard was filled with fireflies. Animals that light up . . . such a thing can stoke a child's wonder. But so can the stars in the sky. Look at them all! You've read about them (or been read to about them), you've heard the nursery rhymes, and now you are beneath them, and you know they are a very long way away. And they have been around for a very long time. And you feel a certain kind of thrill looking at them, something you have never felt before, something that is almost fear but definitely isn't anything to be afraid of, not even when the first of a lifetime's shivers runs up your spine.

Or that time you were with your big brother, when you were both still kids, and it rained so hard every person left the beach, no one as far as the eye could see, and the Atlantic Ocean was roiling in the storm, and the fat raindrops made little craters when they hit the hard-packed sand. The ocean was warm when we entered it to escape the cold rain, and we let ourselves be stirred in the swells and chop, by the whims of the great force, until the storm passed. Yes, it was a thrill, but it was different back then, because that was the only world I knew and I was already part of it.

It is like what David Foster Wallace said in his Kenyon commencement speech about the fish. Two young fish are swimming along and an older fish passes by and asks, "How is the water today?" and after he's gone, one young fish asks the other, "What the hell is water?"

The younger fish were so immersed in their element, they didn't know there was anything else. They hadn't yet learned about the door that can separate us from our deepest experiences.

———————

MY HEART GOT LEFT in a classroom on the campus of the University of Montana on March 17, 2020. By that point I'd had students for more than twenty years. I haven't had one since.

Me falling into teaching was about as unlikely as a child falling into a well. In my early twenties in Chicago I bought suits and wore ties and took the train downtown to this office building or that. My closest friends were accountant, banker, lawyer, trader, lawyer, lawyer, med student, banker. I was the crazy one—my job was in marketing.

In my last semester of college, my Spanish 202 summer-school teacher asked me if I had ever thought about being a teacher. He was about the age my father would have been if he had lived that long. His comment thrilled and insulted me. He was an impressive teacher and his suggestion that I do what he did made me feel like he thought *I* was impressive, too. But I also wondered: Did he think so little of me that he thought the best I could make of myself was to become a teacher? Did he think I didn't have a chance of making it in the "real" world?

Early on in my teaching career, I made the decision to scuttle the timeworn agenda of the administrators and surreptitiously started to teach my seventy-five-minute Lit class as a semester-long argument on why critical thinking is imperative.

On the first day of the semester I'd say something like, "Who gives a flying fuck about literature?" They'd respond by looking around the room at one another, much the way Max looked when I invited him onto the bed. "Is this for real?" they'd be thinking. "He's messing with us, isn't he?" The truth is, I had no right or reason to expect them to care about a class they were taking only because it was required (and were enduring with a fair amount of dread). They were chemistry majors and forestry majors and business majors. I'd be lucky if out of my twenty-five students even two of them were English majors. So why should we go through the same motions that every other miserable Intro to Lit student has gone through for the past zillion years?

Early on I'd ask them if they had ever seen football players at practice jumping through tires that were laid out on the field. My students—especially when I was teaching in Alabama—would perk up any time I mentioned football. "Have you ever seen a running back break into the open, get halfway to the end zone, and then encounter two rows of tires he has to step through right there in the middle of the field?"

My assignments were not to get them to understand literature or appreciate literature. I had them read text simply to high-step through the tires, and then take that skill into the "real" world so that they could read the world as the text it is, a construction of mostly invisible choices that are intended to manipulate the way we think and the way we feel. I told them if they could make that invisible world visible, their world would expand into a vastness, and it would lead them to riches and love, meaning and joy.

IT WAS IN HIGH SCHOOL that I first became aware of the door. At night, while my brother was away at college, I would wait for my mother and father to retire to their bedroom, and then I would slip out of bed, tiptoe around my pitch-black room to find my black sweatpants and black sweatshirt, and then I'd tiptoe down the stairs (avoiding the one near the turn at the bottom that squeaked), and in the kitchen I'd slowly—very slowly—ease open the sliding-glass door, and I'd step out into the night.

In my backyard, not more than ten yards from the house, right in the middle of the lawn—where as a little kid I'd throw the ball up in the air and then look at the window to see if my mother was watching—there was the stump of an old oak tree that had been struck by lightning. I would stride in my bare feet across the dew-moist lawn and squat on that stump. I'd gather wet dirt from around its base and spread it over my feet and hands and then across my face. And then, once I felt invisible, I would run.

In my bare feet, down the asphalt streets, across the moon-silvered lawns, through the wooded areas of backyards, I'd run, for hours at a time, the suburb belonging only to me and my thoughts. Mostly I ran, but sometimes I would stop at the house of a girl who was special to me and I would sit on the bench on her front porch, the same bench where she and I used to sit some nights when my friend and I knocked uninvited on her door. And sometimes I would stretch out on her backyard patio furniture. This all seems strange to me now, but at the time it made total sense. It was necessary, even urgent.

One late-July night I got off the patio chair and slid open the glass door to her house and stepped inside. I didn't roam around or anything. I just stood still in the dark of her living room and felt like I wasn't completely alone in the world. Those were hard years, but the night opened a door and helped me feel normal, hid my skinniness, and revealed the mystery of the world—its bigness, its beauty—and in this world the girl was safely asleep upstairs in her silent house, and for a moment I got to be close to her.

————

MY THERAPIST ASKED ME a few months ago what my favorite part of the day was. I really thought hard about her question. (I'm a good patient.) I try to be honest with my therapist. (I need results.) Have I been honest? I think so, but it's really hard to know if you're truly honest. I mean, how much massaging of the truth do we do? How much do we—especially on an unconscious level—tweak things here or there to make ourselves look better, to make ourselves less culpable, to explain the wrong turns in our life as someone else's fault?

At one point my therapist told me I was too honest. "In relationships," she said, "you don't have to tell the other person everything." For instance, she explained, if you are walking down the street and see a pretty woman, you don't have to point her out to the woman you love. Makes sense to me. But what if the woman I love asks? That's where my therapist said truth massaging was called for.

And there are other opportunities for truth adjustments. For example, if you are struggling with getting old and losing your vitality and youth and beauty and athleticism, maybe that's an issue you should keep to yourself. And if you do have to talk about it, maybe you don't have to talk about *all* of it. You certainly don't have to talk about it in a way that somehow feels threatening to the woman you love, the woman who is also struggling with not being young.

I think what I said to my therapist when she told me all this was something like, "You're a therapist?!"

She thinks truth massaging is a social norm—even in relationships—and it is how you protect people. I think she is nuts.

I said something like, "So I have an issue that is a very common human challenge, and especially so for me, and I am not supposed to explore it with the person I want to spend the rest of my life with?!" And she said, "Exactly. Now you're getting it."

I understand the desire to protect people. But with L. I had arrived at a point where I was ready to leave the trappings of youth behind. I was ready to start the slow drift of "growing old" with her, and I was even ready to do so with excitement. I was confident that I was ready, that everything would be okay.

But my therapist suggested that my honesty could become a weapon, a damage maker, a divider. (I think it's the glue.)

What my therapist said about honesty is a horrifying thought, and it's about the worst thing someone could say to me. My whole goal in relationships is to make safe spaces for the people (and birds) I care about. Like last night, for instance. Last night I had nine birds roaming around my house. Four of them are disabled, three of them are juveniles, and two of them left their parents' nest yesterday.

I slept well with all those birds under my roof. And the next morning I kept the front door closed and felt joy watching them roam about, making their little cooing and *chukking* sounds.

Some were walking across the floor pecking at things, some were flying from perch to perch. My living room looked and sounded like a busy rookery. I could have charged admission. And it was comforting not to feel the knife of loneliness stabbing me in the gut for a change.

It took me a while, but I finally arrived at a real answer for my therapist about what my favorite part of the day is. "The plain and simple fact," I told her, "is the best part of my day is when I am dreaming."

L. IS IN MY DREAMS, and the boy, too. As I mentioned, the boy is always the age he was when he was on the rope swing—almost six—and L. is the same age she was when we bought our house and got engaged to be married. I wonder if the boy still gets that sudden look of delight on his face, the one he had after we ended our sixteenth consecutive game of Trouble and we looked at each other and at the same time said, "One more?"

The odd thing about my dreams is that my dream-self is never in pain. Isn't that strange? Why, in the four years since I landed in that hospital in Kuala Lumpur, has my dream-self never once been afflicted? My dream-self's life is full of adventures and intimacy, and he is hopeful about the future. My dream-self is not disabled. He plays hockey and throws the baseball and bicycles up hillsides. He chases after people on the pitch and gets chased by people who want to kill him with knives. He can fly. So of course my dreams are the best part of my day.

The mornings when I wake up and I don't remember any intensely pleasurable dreams—those moments make me feel like I am in for a long day. I guess this is what it means to get up on the wrong side of the bed. On those days, the clock becomes my enemy. (Even more so than usual.) I have to kill fifteen hours or so of my mostly joyless waking life while being in unending pain before I get another chance to experience the intense joy that comes to me when I am in my world of dreams.

MY LEGS WENT WEAK last weekend for some unknown reason. In the shower—when I managed to take one—they were all trembly and I was worried I'd fall down, reaching out at the last moment for the shower curtain before pulling it down with me like soon-to-be-dead characters do in slasher movies.

And then the migraine hit. By sheer happenstance, this was the same day my pain reprocessing therapist informed me that we had "hit a wall" and that our time together had reached its end. The "wall" she was referring to was my ME/CFS. She said, "I'm not doing my job if I only reduce your pain but fail to improve your functionality."

Her reasoning was that true improvement in quality of life comes from functioning. Exercise and activity are good for most of the chronic-pain people she works with. So she first uses mindfulness/neuroplasticity tricks to reduce the pain, then she nudges her patients to take advantage of it. Go for a walk! Take a trip! Play Frisbee golf! Those things sound incredible.

But activity/exertion—any expenditure that goes beyond one's "energy envelope"—is bad for people like me, possibly catastrophic. This fact was illustrated in the worst possible way when a reputable medical journal, *The Lancet*, published a "study" that proved that graded exercise therapy (GET) was very beneficial for ME/CFS patients. As a result, some ME/CFS patients who had been suffering for years or decades decided to try GET (even though it went against everything their bodies were telling them). Doctors said, "Keep pushing." (In other words, stay on the upward "grade" of exercise.) The result was that many of

Buckbee & Fitzgerald

those desperate people "crashed," and crashed hard. Many of them never left the house again. Some never left the couch. A few never left their beds. And many of them decided to leave the earth.

It took years for *The Lancet* to retract their article. Maybe they didn't believe ME/CFS was a real disease.

So I told my PRT, "Just because I feel less pain doesn't mean I should be more active." She looked at me quizzically, like I had said the medical equivalent of "The earth is flat."

"In fact," I added, "in a way you are setting a trap. Because with my pain down, I may feel inclined to do more." She looked at me as if to say, "And?" Like, that was the whole point of the work we were doing. I'm not sure she believes ME/CFS is a real illness, either.

My brother kept nudging me to travel or move. I told him I thought the energy required for either one would make me sicker. But he kept bringing it up. I think my brother may doubt that ME/CFS is real, too.

I can't tell you how many times in the past four years I pushed myself beyond my energy envelope (essentially doing GET) before I heard the ME/CFS experts nix GET. The result of all those attempts wasn't just pain and frustration, but I also felt like a failure. I felt weak. And pathetic. I was quite sure most of my doctors, and friends, and family thought so, too.

———

TODAY IS HALLOWEEN, the one day of the year you get to be somebody else. But I want to be somebody else every day. (I want to be who I was.) Maybe I could carry a hockey stick or a piece of chalk or a flower meant for someone special. But I can't seem to get away from who I am, so there's not much to celebrate.

I realize I have sounded kind of miserable lately, and there's a reason for that. (It's because I've been kind of miserable lately.) But I'm thinking people may not like this side of me so much. I may be more likable when I am feeling the world's beauty and making friends with a bird while an undercurrent of hopefulness flows beneath it all.

Halloween is also an anniversary of sorts. This is the anniversary of the day my illness really began, four years ago. (It feels like fifty.)

It was several years after L. left me, and I'd tried to move on (I even had some romantic relationships), but clearly I had more suffering to do. I started thinking that maybe a journey to a distant place would help.

The analogy that came to mind was the forty-days-and-forty-nights kind of thing. Like biblical characters in a desert. Go in in turmoil; come out in peace. Sure, you'll get physically battered—sun, dehydration, vultures, locusts—but that's just the price you have to pay.

Instead of the desert, I chose Southeast Asia again. And instead of forty days, I chose five months. I planned to explore new and familiar destinations. I was definitely going to Bali, maybe Railay in Thailand (where I saw the bats and collapsed), and a few remote islands. Borneo, with its ancient rainforests and rare orangutans, was my ultimate destination. It was as close to wild as I might ever get on this planet.

I had no map because I had no plan. I was coordinating around earthquakes, the rainy seasons, and my state of mind in any given moment. I knew I was going to be alone, for a long time, and I was going to carry my grief with me everywhere I went. I'd steer into the suffering, but I'd also, when desperate, steer a little bit away. I planned the trip for months, and for months I dreaded the entire escapade.

When I arrived in Bali in October of 2018, I quickly moved to the quiet north shore. In Pemuteran, I rented a fancy ($26 a night!) bungalow with a comfortable bed that was draped with holeless mosquito netting. In the middle of my first night in Pemuteran I woke up because my room was shaking. "Oh," I realized, "this is what an earthquake feels like."

The tremors were violent enough to shake objects off the shelves and to make you feel unsteady—or at least uneasy—on your feet. I went outside and heard a few voices carrying across the dark grounds, but nobody seemed concerned. The staff didn't knock on doors and the few guests who were staying there didn't come out to talk about the excitement or what to do next.

We were on a bay that was surrounded by hillsides on an island in the middle of an ocean, and we seemed to be ideally situated to be wiped out by a tsunami—tourists, staff, fishermen, and the fishermen's chickens, too. But nobody was evacuating, and the hillsides were too far away to scamper up, so I decided to go back to my bungalow. Not much later, though, the alarms went off, maybe amplified by the same speakers that played the daily calls to prayer. I grabbed my headlamp and headed over to the palapa bar, where I thought I would be most likely to see a gathering of people. But, again, there were no guests, and the only staff were two security guards. They didn't act worried at all. In fact, they seemed annoyed. I hung out with them for a while anyway, staring at the bay to see if the black waters were retreating, and after an hour or so, when nothing happened, I went back to bed. I later found out that what I thought was an earthquake was an aftershock to the main event, which had happened two weeks earlier and which measured 7.5 and triggered a tsunami. Though the tsunami didn't reach Bali, the places it did reach were devastated, and thousands of people died.

Each morning in Pemuteran, I would walk with my snorkeling gear down the black-sand beach, weaving my way through the fishermen's boats and the fishermen's chickens, and I would enter the water. In the sand-bottomed shallows, I was greeted by the same seahorse every time. He was always alone, gently swaying in the gentle tide, his curled tail sometimes bouncing against the ocean's floor, sometimes finding a piece of seagrass to wrap itself around so he could stay in one place. Seahorses are like pigeons—they mate for life—and I wondered if this guy was waiting for his partner to show up. The male seahorse gives birth to the babies, so maybe he was just killing time in the turquoise sea, waiting for his thousand children to be born.

On that strip of beach I saw the ocean for the first time since losing L., and I entered the ocean for the first time since losing L., and everything I saw for the first time, like that seahorse, reminded me that there was no one by my side who could enjoy it with me.

In the evenings, around the time the call-to-prayer speakers blared, I'd retreat to my bungalow. Sometimes I'd go for a late-evening swim in the pool and then find a comfy cushioned chair in the palapa bar under the palm-thatched roof. The bay, just steps away, was quiet and black, and sometimes I'd swim there in the night, even though the staff or guards always advised against it. They were afraid I'd get hit by one of the small fishermen's boats that trickled into the bay and docked on the beach. But risking a collision with an outboard engine was totally consistent with the forty-days-forty-nights thing, so I mostly ignored them.

Later I'd have room service delivered to me—usually some kind of fish (which I felt bad about, seeing as they had provided me so much joy when I was snorkeling with them), a bottle of Bintang, and a small fried-banana ice cream sundae for dessert.

I wasn't getting much social interaction, so one day I signed up to learn how to scuba dive. The instructor asked me if I wanted to get into the pool, and I said, "Can't we do it in the ocean?" He asked me if I was a good swimmer. I told him I once swam ten miles in the ocean, and that seemed to be enough to convince him.

We headed out on a small boat with a dozen or so snorkelers, and on the way, while talking loudly over the sounds of the hull slapping the water and the saltwater breeze, he showed me the gear and taught me hand signals and figured out how much weight to put in my dive belt and suited me up.

The boat anchored in a small channel and the snorkelers jumped off the boat and dispersed, their heads buried in the sea like the helpless prey of some mythical creature. There was a decent amount of wind that day, and it chopped up the ocean, and I was glad that I would be in the relative calm below, free from the motion sickness that came while bobbing on the surface.

I sat on the edge of the boat and tipped backwards, like real scuba divers do in the movies, and I turned and twisted in the water until I was seated on the sand bottom as I'd been instructed. My instructor then sat across from me and we began going through the lesson—hand signals, losing and finding the regulator, sharing a regulator, checking gauges, etc.

We were only in about eight feet of water, but the problem was the current. The wind was now combining with the shifting tide, and not only couldn't I stay in a seated position, but I also started bumping off corals and drifting along the bottom away from the boat (and my instructor). He tried to physically wrangle me back to my spot, but because we were in a channel, the current further intensified, at which point my instructor had to let me go. When we surfaced, he was clearly worried. Apparently, these conditions were "extreme" for a person who has never even scuba dived in a pool before. He shouted at me to just allow myself to drift, and so I went with the flow, and he did, too, staying by my side, and in what felt like seconds we were more than a half mile from the boat.

My instructor and I continued to drift. "It's okay," I kept telling him. "It's no problem." And it really wasn't. Perhaps my confidence in the water was unwarranted, but I was pretty much enjoying the whole adventure. Though it may have been an illegal, unethical, and perhaps even immoral way to teach a beginner, for me it was perfect.

The next diving mecca I visited was Tulamben, where the instructor was aghast when I told him about my experience in Pemuteran and insisted I give him the name of the irresponsible instructor and the dive shop. I lied and told him I couldn't remember.

The Tulamben dive location was about seventy miles to the east, and the highlight there was a wreck called the USS *Liberty*, a cargo ship that had been torpedoed by the Japanese navy in 1942 and towed to shore. It sat on the beach for a couple of decades until the nearby volcano erupted, shaking the earth enough to slide the *Liberty* into the sea.

That dive was much easier, perhaps in part because my instructor insisted that I practice in the pool before we entered the ocean. The hardest part for me was maintaining a consistent depth. I would rise or sink, and my instructor would grab me and reorient me. I'd say the experience was jaw-dropping, but of course dropping my jaw would have caused me to lose my regulator's mouthpiece and drown, so instead I'll just say this: a lot of doors opened. There were soft corals and hard corals of all colors, including fan corals that looked about as wide as I am tall. We swam through scattering damsels and schools of jackfish, poked our heads into holes in the wreck that were home to giant grouper, and were passed by a number of turtles (who seemed to have no problem at all maintaining the proper depth). The highlight, though, by far, was a creature called a "garden eel."

In many ways, the garden eel is just an ordinary eel, but what makes it extraordinary and turns it into a skilled door-opener is how it hides from predators. When threatened, the garden eel, which is about two feet long, anchors its tail to the sandy floor and holds its body in a vertical position. Put fifty garden eels together and they look identical to a field of seagrass, swaying gently in the underwater current the same way seagrass does. When startled, the eels all at once drop straight down into their holes and vanish. In the blink of an eye, the field is gone. But when they sense the coast is clear, they rise straight up, out of their holes, and resume their imitation of a plant no fish-eating fish would give a second look.

IN OTHER PARTS of the country, winter may officially start at the end of December, but here in Missoula, it starts today. We are only a few days into November, and all the pigeons in the flock are desperate to get in my house. They hang around until the late afternoon, waiting for me to soften up and let them in. I expect at some point I will, and then I will have forty birds spending the night in my kitchen.

AFTER MY DIVE IN TULAMBEN, I had dinner at a beachside hotel restaurant. The view was terrific, but the fish tasted a little funky. My table was on the nearly empty second-floor patio, from where I could see the top part of the smoking volcano, which was maybe fifteen or so miles away. If you ever read in the news about air traffic being denied over Bali, or restrictions on tourists, it's because of Mount Agung. The same eruption that caused the *Liberty* to slide into the ocean also killed hundreds of people. I thought about the end of *Joe Versus the Volcano*, how just when Joe is about to jump into the smoking volcano, he is joined by Patricia, the woman he loves. She tells him that she loves him and says, "I've never been in love before."

In response, Joe says that he has never been in love before, either.

Looking at the volcano in Tulamben that evening, I couldn't help but think about watching *Joe Versus the Volcano* with L. snuggled beside me.

After dinner, I sat on the cement break wall with a sweating bottle of beer between my legs, looking out at the quiet ocean. The sun set and the sky darkened. The palapa bar was empty. When I was ready for my second Bintang, I told the bartender I'd buy one for him if he wanted to join me. Imported taxes make beer expensive in Bali—a single beer is as expensive as the meal itself. He retrieved a couple of cold bottles from the bar and took a seat next to me on the cement wall, and we talked about what life in Bali was like and how his family survived the earthquake in Lombok the previous year.

My thoughts drifted after he left. Up the beach I saw the silhouettes of a group of people. Or were they creatures from the Black Lagoon? I couldn't tell. They lined up single file, turned on their headlamps, and took hold of a rope that was anchored high up the shore. Then they slowly began walking into the ocean. But their movements were awkward, and I realized it was because they were walking backwards, which meant they were wearing flippers and were about to do a night dive around the wreck.

I've swum far out into the Atlantic Ocean at night, and I have swum far out into the Pacific at night, and, as I mentioned, I swam far out into a frigid Lake Michigan at night, but I had never swum deep *down* inside the ocean at night. I decided this was something I would have to do before I returned home. I wanted to stand on the bottom of the ocean, a hundred feet down, and see if I could summon up a craving for the wondrous turmoil that awaited me above the surface.

LATER THAT NIGHT, I woke up from a fever dream, sweating, intensely nauseous, and I knew what that meant. I started a mental stopwatch in my mind and began a fifteen-hour countdown, which is how long it normally takes for this particular misery to pass. I was in the desert now, for sure, and the plagues had been set loose.

At one point, between sprints to the bathroom, I was curled up in the tiny bed in the fetal position and saw a good-sized rat scuttling along the tile floor, hugging the wall, until it disappeared under the door of my room. I fell asleep briefly, then woke up with that sickening urgency again. Before crawling back to bed, I thought about stuffing some towels into the gap beneath the door. But I didn't know if by doing so I would end up keeping the rat out or trapping him in. Was there a part of me that would have preferred that the rat be locked in the room with me? Absolutely! The suffering had come, and I was ready to steer into it.

The next morning I had to get up early in order to cancel the dive I'd scheduled. This was especially disappointing because I had a waterproof postcard prepared to send to my writing mentor. Tulamben is noted for having the only underwater postal box in the world, and my mentor had been working on some kind of mysterious postcard project for years, sending out hundreds of them to former students and colleagues and who-knows-who-else, and then getting some in return. I sure would have liked to add my underwater postcard with the Bali postmark to his mounting collection. I bet he didn't have one of those. I promised myself I would come back to Tulamben before leaving Bali, so I could go for a dive and drop him that postcard.

Surprisingly, I didn't feel that bad, even though I was well short of the fifteen-hour mark. I checked in with my body and couldn't hear a stopwatch ticking at all. I still wasn't up for a dive, but I grabbed my snorkeling gear and walked down the hill to the stone beach. I slid into the water and explored the shallows, then headed over to the wreck and hovered above it for a while. Even though the water was clear, I couldn't see far enough down to spot the garden of eels swaying in the current, or the groupers hiding in their holes, or whatever other mysteries you have to get right up next to in order to see, like the clownfish hiding in the anemones and the tiny scorpionfish that are camouflaged to blend in with the coral.

The next morning I hired a car and left Tulamben, and the volcano, and the wreck, and the rat.

I never made it back there. I didn't get to see the garden of eels again, and I never got to do a night dive, and my mentor never got to go to his mailbox and find inside it a waterproof postcard that had been dropped in a postal box anchored to the bottom of an ocean on the other side of the world from a former student who loved him.

I drove to a busy port town in the southeast part of Bali and bought a ticket for a ferry that would take me to a small island about forty minutes away. It wasn't scheduled to leave for hours, but afraid I'd miss a departure or screw something else up somehow, I got to the dock way too early. There were a few other ticketed passengers milling about, but it was mostly calm and quiet. I bought a Coke and some Pringles from a local vendor and used my gigantic duffel as a beanbag chair and watched some laughing little kids playing in the kind-of-dirty water.

———

WHILE I WAS WAITING for my ferry to show up, a ferry from Lombok arrived. Lombok was the island that had the big earthquake the year before, but because the entire livelihood of the people of Lombok was dependent on tourism, they reopened amid the rubble.

Lombok was about two hours by ferry from Bali. The crossing must have been rough that day, because the people stumbling off the ferry did not look good *at all*. They were unsteady on their feet, their faces ashen. I asked one girl what happened, and without breaking stride, she murmured, "Everyone got sick." Dozens of passengers hurried past me, as if desperate to get their feet on solid ground.

That was enough to get me to really start worrying about my own trip. I've always had a phobia of getting sick in public, and though I may not have had a "weak" stomach, it certainly was inconsistent. I could endure choppy seas on a small boat one day and then get carsick while in the driver's seat the next. To add to my anxiety that day, the skies were darkening and there were ominous patches far out over the ocean where it was pouring rain.

The ferry that pulled up to the jetty looked bloated and slow and old, as if its next phase of life (as a wreck beneath the sea where ocean critters would dwell) was not too far off.

The skies continued to darken, especially out over the ocean in the same direction we were heading. Finally, we were allowed to board, and everyone scrambled to get in line so they could get on first. Most of them rushed into the hold below, which surprised me. I've always preferred to be in the open air, perhaps with a railing to puke over into the ocean, if need be, and if I got wet, so be it, this is life in the tropics. On the top deck were a handful of cheap plastic benches, and that was perfect for me.

IT SNOWED LAST NIGHT. The clocks rolled back. Spring is an hour further away than it was at this time yesterday. My migraine is bad. I need to be on that boat in Bali right now.

THE SUN WASN'T OUT, at least not at first. I waited for the water to get rougher as we got farther from the shore, but clearly our stretch of ocean was calmer than the one from Lombok. It drizzled, not unpleasantly in the sticky heat, but we steered clear of the downpours. The handful of passengers on the top deck with me seemed to be enjoying the elements, and I grabbed on to the coattails of their calm.

The ferry took us to a floating dock in the calm waters of a channel between two islands. Nobody knew what was going on, and some of the tourists began asking a lot of questions and producing a lot of anxiety.

I found a quiet place to sit on the dock and dangled my legs over the edge. The sun was coming out now, and the sky was blue. Some of the tourists had been traveling for a day or two, and they looked exhausted and frazzled. I imagined how happy they would soon be when they checked into their hotel rooms and collapsed on comfortable beds with linens and pillows, next to mini-fridges that were stocked with Sprites and Cokes and Bintangs.

Eventually, some small boats began pulling up to take us to our different islands. My boat came last, and I found a place on the bench at the back so that I could ride facing forward. A mother and daughter I had struck up a conversation with on the dock offered to take my picture, and I accepted, and today I am so glad I have that picture. I look at it now and I can't believe the person in that photo is me. I look happy in the picture . . . I guess I had taken a reprieve from the forty-days-of-suffering thing. In fact, I felt as if I had left something behind, the weight of loss and worry.

I think now about all the people around me whose lives will someday turn on a dime (for the worse). How unsuspecting they are. It's hard to see the dime when the small boat you're on splashes up ocean spray, and everyone gets soaked and laughs.

For a moment there is such joyful camaraderie around the shared experience of the world's beauty and wonder.

When I talk about my travels, I feel like I can breathe, like I am using a part of my lungs I haven't used in a long time. But for the most part, I was a fucking wreck in Bali. If divers were to explore the wreck that was me, they would surface and remove their mouthpieces, and a movie-star-looking man with salt water dripping off his short beard would say, "Wow, that was a lot of damage." And in reply, a young woman with manicured eyebrows and an Italian accent would say, "Yes, it was, and now there are all those other living creatures moving in and hiding inside him, living in a thing that no longer lives."

Right now, I'm at a table in the middle of the coffee shop, surrounded by conversation, enduring the slithering headache while polishing the story I dictated to my computer this morn-ing, trying not to go home. Everyone here is with someone else. A small towheaded child just came in wearing a puffy coat that looks bigger than he is.

Every child I see is the boy.

———

THE WHEELS REALLY BEGAN to fall off on that tiny yoga-retreat island, Nusa Lembongan. The island was small enough to walk from one end to the other, and I did that, in the oppressive heat, repeatedly. On the north end was a mangrove bay with a couple of tiki-type bars on the beach. I'd walk up the quiet road with my snorkeling gear, and when people on motorbikes or in cars would slow down and offer me a ride, I'd decline. At the mangroves, I'd slip on my fins, mask, and snorkel and slide into the water.

The reef was about a quarter mile out, and I usually beat the tourist boats to it, but eventually they'd appear, and dozens of life-preserved snorkelers would bob in the shallows with me, staring down at the brain coral and butterfly fish and tangs and puffers. I'd dive as deep as I could, but the bottom was rarely more than fifteen feet below. Occasionally, I'd climb aboard one of the tour boats and sit next to the other tired snorkelers (who had actually bought tickets for the boat) and we'd talk about the marvels we'd seen. Then I'd jump back in the water and snorkel some more before I climbed aboard another tour boat to talk to some more tourists. The tour guides didn't know I didn't belong, or they didn't care. Hours later, I'd swim back to shore, keeping my body flat when I reached the shallow water so I could beach myself USS *Liberty*-style on the hot sand.

I'd warm myself in the sun—it wouldn't take long—and head to one of the ramshackle bars to buy a Coke, drinking it in the shade while staring at the sea. Then I'd follow the curve of the beach back to my hotel.

At the south end of the island was a popular bar on a cliff overlooking a rough-water beach. Many tourists come here to visit a spot called "Devil's Tears," where the thundering waves produce large clouds of misty spray filled with rainbows of light. It's a great place to get a selfie or two, though a number of people have been swept into the ocean by roguish waves, dying in their attempt to capture how wonderful their life is.

Near sunset, after the tour groups departed, I would find a rock ledge to sit on and watch the crashing waves make storms and rainbows. One evening I met a German girl who tried to talk me into going on a motorbike ride with her. I asked, "How long have you been riding a motorbike?" And she said, "A few days."

When you are in any tourist area in Southeast Asia, you can close your eyes and throw a dart and hit a Western tourist who has been mangled in a motorbike accident. If you were in the gauze-and-crutches business in Thailand or Bali, you could make a fortune on those misfortunes. Though I would have liked to sit behind the German girl and wrap my arms around her, I declined, even though she was rather striking and could have relieved me of the many-miles walk back to my hotel.

But I was suffering now, sweating out the loss and grief, and so I walked. And I walked. In the daytime and at night, wearing my jeans and a long-sleeve shirt. And I swam. Out to the reef mostly, but sometimes up and down the coast. And as my body wore down and I got tired and my sleep was disturbed by small doses of what I later would learn was post-exertional malaise, my response was to walk more, swim more.

I was on an island that was teeming with lovely young yoga students, but that only made me feel more alone. One night while walking up the main road after dinner, a few girls dashed across the street toward me. They were in a panic, yelling about some psycho who was stalking them. They were fairly young, in their early twenties, I guess. They were genuinely frightened, but also kind of excited at the same time. I don't know why I looked safe to them—it may have been that they were in a hurry to tell someone, anyone, about the little far-from-home adventure they were having. They told me all about their run-ins with this guy, and I walked them back to their hotel. "If I see him," I told them before we parted, "I'll beat him up for you." They didn't realize I was joking and interpreted my comment as a gesture of gallantry, which was fine with me, seeing as there was no burning bus around to save them from.

This island was a place L. and I had decided to visit at some point after we married. We were going to take a marathon trip together. Joe and Patricia in *Joe Versus the Volcano* end the movie by saying they want to "get away from the things of man." I suppose that's kind of what we were fantasizing about, the "things of man" being all the outside pressures we were weathering together. But it seems she had some other thoughts running at the same time beneath the surface, just far enough down so I couldn't see them. Because I now know if I dove down and swam through them—those other thoughts of hers—that current of water would have felt very, very cold.

———

I SPENT ABOUT A WEEK on that island before I moved to an even smaller island, where I stayed at an expat's hotel/resort. My bungalow was near the edge of a cliff that overlooked the ocean. There was a real communal feel to the place, but no one seemed very interested in me. I stretched out in the oversized lounge furniture by the saltwater pool, drinking Heinekens and reading tattered paperback books that previous guests had left behind. Those were the last books I ever read (it was the last time I was able to read books), in the fading light of sunset on that clifftop below which surfers rode the orange- and red-streaked waves.

I listen to books sometimes now, but it's not the same. I miss the feel of a book in my hand, the rustle of pages turning. I've tried to read in the past few years, but the way it forces my eyes to move back and forth seems to always blow up my headache. (I'm not even reading right now! I know my story so well that when I polish it I don't have to look that close or that long at the screen. I can skip around or skip altogether.)

I shouldn't have started talking about my headache. Now it's on the top of my mind (literally), so I better call it quits. It's hard to leave the coffee shop—even though it's a hive of noisy activity—because I know I won't see another person (at least not a three-dimensional one) for the rest of the day. But I've got birds at home. Two babies I call "the twins" are probably huddling together, maybe grooming the back of each other's necks. The other birds are pecking at the kitchen floor or resting in a beam of sun, and I'll take my place among them.

———

MY EDITOR HAS VANISHED on me. I haven't heard from her in a week, and we were maybe supposed to talk a few days ago. In an email last weekend, I asked her whether I should keep talking about my tour around Asia. My rambling seemed pointless and random to me, and so I told her I would wait to hear from her before dictating anything more. Days went by, and I heard not a peep (as my mother used to say).

Previously, I was sending her a chunk of "polished" dictation just about every day, and just about every day she'd read it and respond with words of praise and encouragement. She's a very generous person, quite kind, and I also trust her opinions. She made me believe my trip around Bali matters.

But when I didn't hear from her, the doubt crept back in: "I'm wasting my time. This serves no purpose. I have a purposeless life (except for my birds)." And the story began to disappear. I felt at sea, as if I was drifting farther and farther away from the shores of Bali, and the islands were fading in the mist.

For some unexpected reason, talking about my trip has made me feel like I am back in Southeast Asia. Telling the story of my travels is not the same as being there, of course. I think maybe retellings of life events like that have a half-life. So I am experiencing some intensity and richness (fear and beauty and door-openings), but it is only half of what it was when I was actually there. And if I ever do tell this story again, the half-life will again be cut in half. The intensity is dissolving, dissipating, like salt in the ocean. It has barely enough buoyancy to keep me afloat.

I haven't told the story about my trip to Asia before. By the time I did make it back to the States, I was too sick to share it. Just thinking about trying to string coherent sentences together was enough to give me a migraine (or make my migraine worse). Days slipped by, and then weeks, and then my trip was old news. And I didn't really have anyone to tell it to anyway. The only people I was mumbling semi-coherently to were doctors and nurses and receptionists. Unlike the neurologist and my GP and the gastro, the infectious disease doctor at least wanted to know some details about my journey. I remember sitting in the examination room under the fluorescent lights in excruciating pain, my eyes mostly closed, answering his questions about where I went and what I ate and what symptoms I was displaying. But despite the pain I was feeling under those flickering lights (and fluorescent lights are *always* flickering to people in migraine), I made a point of throwing in an irrelevant detail here and there, so my experience of those few months wasn't completely erased, didn't disappear to the bottom of a deep, dark ocean. I told him things like, "I spent a lot of time scuba diving around a field of garden eels . . . *but* while doing so I was sharing communal scuba equipment, mouth-pieces and such." Or: "In the evenings, after watching the sun set over the rough-surf ocean, I'd walk back to my hotel through the street-food markets . . . *but* I'd stop under a tree and stare up at the many bats that were mingling among the low branches."

I was confident the infectious disease doctor was going to solve my health problem. I was sure that whatever had gone wrong with me had to do with some food I ate or the bats I stood under or the giant rat that was in my room in Tulamben.

I know I will never get to go back to Asia. My favorite places in the world—the places I was supposed to go to with the woman I loved—are cut off from me forever. This, right now, as the snow falls and I sit on my couch and talk to my computer, is as close as I will get to Pemuteran or the *Liberty* wreck or Devil's Tears. When I get done talking about these things, those places, I know I won't ever get close to them again.

———

IT'S DOWNRIGHT FRIGID OUTSIDE, and my physical capacity is next to nil. Two rooms of my tiny house are my lifeboat—the kitchen and living room, which are basically one room. In movies, when a sailor is stranded at sea, a seagull inevitably lands on his lifeboat, and then the shipwrecked sailor does all he can to kill it. Those scenes have always disturbed me, not because it isn't rational for a dying man to bludgeon a bird with an oar so he can eat it raw, but because the filmmakers never seem to emphasize the awe a person like that might feel. (Joe would have felt it.) If you are nearing your exit from this world, and its beauty and wonder is presented to you one last time—in the form of a creature that can fly (!), and has been around forever, and can drink salt water (salt water!)—wouldn't you put your desperation aside, if only for a second, and marvel at the bigness of it all? Wouldn't you think, maybe it's *not* worth killing?

I don't have seagulls on my living room life raft, but I have a whole lot of pigeons. At last count, there were nine of them. They are mostly still and quiet, but from time to time something stirs them to action all at once, and they fly from perch to perch and room to room, looking much like a flock of seagulls that has chanced upon a school of herring, and at such times I can almost feel the aimless drift of the ocean and the couch rocking in the waves.

———

I HAVEN'T SEEN V. in a week, but at least my editor returned. (Her mother, the one who loved to travel the world, who took Carol Ann to Russia, passed away. Carol Ann is heartbroken but insists this story is helping her get through it.) The last time I saw V. she was in the nesting box with Two-Step, eating birdseed from their bowl. But last Wednesday, when I was walking up my cracked cement-track driveway, I watched Two-Step take off from his perch on the light post and glide straight at me. He flew so gracefully, so effortlessly—he's really come a long way. Just like in the old days, he landed square on the top of my head.

He even stayed on my head as I walked toward the house, and he probably wouldn't have jumped off at all, except I stopped under their window box and coaxed him off. He flapped up to the diving-board entrance and pushed his head through the entrance-cover curtain and disappeared.

Later that night, when I heard him chortling, I stood up on my coffee table and poked open the venetian-blind slats to check on him and V., and she wasn't there. Two-Step was alone, looking into the living room, his beak pressed right up against the glass pane of the window.

I don't know what has become of V. There are three possibilities. One is that she has decided to find another location that makes for a better nest. That would make sense, because that hungry squirrel has been squeezing into the nesting box again. A second possibility is that she and Two-Step have split up. This would be unusual for pigeons (because pigeons pair up for life). But Two-Step is not an ordinary pigeon, so I'm not sure the typical rules apply to him. It may be that she wanted to move on, but he didn't. Maybe he wanted to stay close to where he raised so many children, and maybe he wanted to stick with the plan they had committed to together. Maybe she never even gave him a clue that she wanted to leave.

The third possibility, of course, is that she is dead.

Whatever the reason, Two-Step doesn't seem very distressed. He's not moping around or anything like that. He's as feisty and territorial as ever, chortling at the other birds, stamping his feet, and puffing out his chest. I can only marvel at his resilience. (And he has only been without her for seven days!)

As a result of V.'s disappearance, I have begun opening the window at nighttime so Two-Step can come into the living room. Does this capitulation represent a total caving in on my part? Absolutely.

Chaos follows Two-Step when he comes inside. The equilibrium the other nine birds have established is disturbed all at once. Two-Step begins claiming every perch, chasing the other birds, and soon they are all flying around like those seagulls I was talking about earlier. The insanity ends when Two-Step settles on a place to perch. If he settles on the ceiling-fan blade in the kitchen, then all the other birds come into the living room; and if he settles on one of the perches in the living room, all the other birds move into the kitchen. Sometimes there are fights, but Two-Step always wins. His beak is always the beak that finds the back of the neck of the bird he's going up against. There is a lot of flapping of wings and the frantic sounds of a bird in crisis. I break up some of the fights, but as soon as I sit back down, they're at it again. (This must have been how my parents felt raising me and my brother.)

Have I raised a bully? I remember back when I started trying to release Two-Step under the pigeon bridge, he would fly up into the rafters and promptly get harassed by a mean bully-bird. That bully would chase Two-Step from rafter to rafter, squawking at him all the while, until Two-Step gave up on trying to fit in with the other birds and returned to my head.

But is he the bully now? I'm hoping that in a few days the birds in my house will get used to one another, and we can have peaceful evenings again, and I can feel calm watching them settle into their comfy resting places, even as I continue to worry in the back of my mind that something terrible has happened to V.

For the moment, as I dictate this on my couch, things have settled down. It is dark outside and the birds are glad to be safe and warm in the embrace of night. Two-Step is in the kitchen on top of the rolling cage that houses the injured couple. Two juvenile siblings are pressed up against each other on a sheet by the hearth. Occasionally, they take turns grooming one another's necks and earholes with their beaks. My spraddle-legged bird is on the floor on a different sheet, one with a paisley print, and I think he thinks he is camouflaged there. And there are other birds, but I can't see them right now. One may be under the coffee table tucked between my boots. Others may be hiding behind the hefty river rocks that line the top of the shelf behind me. Oh, there's a bird! It's the juvenile with the broken wing. He was hiding in plain sight, lying beneath the TV on the soundbar. The soundbar isn't covered with a sheet, but at this point I don't care anymore. You can't cover the entire world with a sheet.

I think my friends would be appalled if they saw my house. I think they would sit me down to "have a talking to." I think after talking to me, they would leave my house and go home and tell their partners that Brian is in real trouble. But what I'm doing makes as much sense as anything else. I have a raging headache, I'm getting skinnier by the day, and there is no land in sight. What do I care if I am surrounded by bird filth? It means, at least, that I am surrounded by birds.

Would L. understand this choice that I am making, the condition of my house? I like to think: Of course so! L. would take pleasure from this sight, feathers floating in the air when the heat comes through the registers, birds lofting and landing. And what if she were in my place on the couch, but with my lap beneath her? Wouldn't that make the pleasure even greater? Wouldn't doors open as we floated far from the things of man on our couch-raft, laughing as we allowed these winged creatures to invite the mystery of the universe into our lives?

———

I HOPE V. IS somewhere safe. I hope, wherever she is, that she is happy with the choice she made.

Actually, to be honest with you, that may not be completely true. Maybe part of me wants V., wherever she is, to be a little bit miserable as a result of abandoning Two-Step. Maybe I want her heart to be filled to the atrial brims with longing-loving thoughts of him. Maybe I want her heart to feel like an overflowing bushel of apples in an orchard at the end of a fall day.

———

NOW I HAVE ELEVEN BIRDS in the house. I feel like I am a day away from completing a Christmas song. At dusk yesterday, when I slid open my living room window to let Two-Step in, there were two birds in the nesting box. V. had returned! I wonder what she has been doing this past week, the things she has seen, the people she has met.

Two-Step was especially ornery to the other birds last night because he wanted to make sure they stayed away from V. The sounds he made when he was close to her were softer and quieter than usual. His coaxing was seductive. Or it was meant to be. It worked for me, at least.

———

I AM NEARING THE END of the story of my Bali trip. My raft is drifting back to shore, but I don't want to get out. Why is it so hard to let go of everything?

At sunset one evening, I sat on the beach and watched the surfers trying to catch the big waves that formed at the point. One surfer in particular caught my attention. He was an older guy, with shaggy graying hair and a beard to match. Sometimes he would catch the wave, sometimes he would miss it completely, and other times he would mistime his pop-up and would quickly and rather dramatically get thrown off his board. There were about five other guys out there with him, all younger, but he pretty much held his own.

Lots of people gathered on the beach to watch the setting sun. The atmosphere was festive, but everyone seemed to be with someone else, so I sat alone and thought about the woman I loved. There was a hole by my side, and it got bigger as the sun set and the sky darkened. All the surfers got out of the water except for the older guy, who was still catching the waves, like a creature of the sea, beneath the descending curtain of night.

THIS FEELING OF PRECIOUSNESS was growing in me that evening on the Balinese island when I watched the surfer from the clifftop. And it wasn't because I was watching an older man who was raging against the dying of the light, if one can "rage" while gliding a surfboard across the lip of a six-foot wave. I was feeling the preciousness because of the sense that something was wrong inside of me and it was growing. When I looked at that man on his board, what I thought was, "I'm afraid I'll never be able to do something like that again."

When the bar began to thin out, I decided it was time to get myself back to my bungalow. On my way up the cement stairs that ran through the center of the bar, I ran into the old guy, who was walking down the stairs. Salt water was still dripping off his shaggy, mostly gray beard, and he had a jaunty giddy-up to his step. This run-in seemed fortuitous because I wanted to tell him how much I enjoyed watching him surf. "You looked pretty good out there," I said. "You caught some of them, and you missed some." I offered to buy him a beer, but he declined.

I suddenly didn't feel ready to leave, because I needed to cling to whatever was left of that day. So I ordered another bottle of beer and retreated back to my place on the edge of the overlook. Now there were no surfers to watch, just one wave after the next, pounding and shaping the shore, one little bit at a time, as they had been doing for eons.

At some point my reverie was broken by the old guy. "If the offer is still good," he said, "I'll take you up on that beer." So I went to the bar and got him a Bintang, and we sat down and started a conversation. He was from Australia, successful in his professional career, and he'd been traveling with a group of guys for years seeking out off-the-beaten-path surf spots. He was smart and engaging and the kind of guy who after about two seconds everyone wants to be.

I told him I was interested in learning to surf. I'd done it once, on my previous trip to Bali, but I had a lot to learn before I could surf a spot like the one beneath that cliff. "Not as much as you'd think," he said, "if you're a half-decent athlete." And then he told me about a good left-breaker where I could practice. What he described sounded great to me, but in the back of my mind I was also thinking about how tired it would make me. The wave was out at the reef, maybe a half mile from shore. And when you first learn to surf you have to use a big board, and the board is so very heavy. And to catch a wave you have to get on your belly and do this awkward wide-armed swim stroke. (Awkward even for someone who had swum hundreds and hundreds of miles.) He talked about surfing, and I got excited, but I felt sick at the same time just thinking about the long swim out to the reef. And this moment, talking to the youthful aging surfer, became yet another instance of my sense that the world, my world, was getting smaller.

A FEW DAYS LATER I went to the beach village where the ferryboats gathered to take people to mainland Bali. The boats backed right up to the shore, where they were tied to stakes on the beach by thick, heavy ropes. Whenever new boats came in, people would rush to the beach to stand in line to board the boat they were ticketed on. The entire scene was a bizarre free-for-all, especially due to the sizable number of tourists who were clumsily wheeling enormous suitcases through the sand, as well as the many languages that were being spoken all at once (and for the most part, not understood). Most of the boat workers spoke Balinese (and only Balinese); most of the tourists were Chinese (and spoke only a dialect of Chinese); and most of the rest of us—even the Germans, French, Dutch, etc.—spoke English, and we all wanted help or information from the others, but our tongues kept us apart.

I was trying to figure out how not to screw up when I spotted my surfer friend. He seemed unfazed by the chaos, and as it turned out we were ticketed on the same boat, so he told me he'd give me a heads-up when our boat arrived and it was time to board.

The only way to get to the boats was to wade through the water. People clearly weren't prepared for this, and they scrambled to get their shoes off and hold on to them while carrying their suitcases above their heads. After giving their suitcases to a deckhand, they had to climb up a swaying ladder to get aboard, which proved to be a challenge for some of the older people, and was, at times, harrowing to watch.

I kept an eye on my surfer friend and watched the scene unfold from the shade of a beachside bar patio while I sipped on yet another Coke. Some of the people who were dragging their bags behind them were tripping on the ropes, which were harmless when they were lying flat on the sand, but which would rise suddenly to about thigh height when the boats they were attached to got pulled out to sea. The wave action would then push the boats back toward shore, and the ropes would go limp and lie harmless and flat, and then the water would recede, pulling the boats, and again the ropes would all pop up at once, tripping more victims.

It was a travel day, and that meant I was wearing jeans and a loose-fitting long-sleeve shirt. When my surfer friend signaled to me that our boat had arrived, I waited for everybody else to board, then joined what was left of the line. I rolled up my pants and carried my shoes—socks stuffed inside—in my free hand. When I got to the boat's ladder, I hoisted my giant duffel up to a deckhand, and he undelicately tossed it on the luggage mountain. There was no deck on this boat, and there wasn't a stern or bow to hang out on either, so the only option was the cabin, which had sixty or so seats.

I immediately found a spot by the entryway where I could stand. Though I was only a few feet away from the five enormous outboard engines and their noxious petrol fumes, I was nearly "outside" in the open air, and there was a refreshing cross breeze. The vibration from the engines was even a bit soothing, and I had a pole to rest against, and I closed my eyes and decided the whole experience was really rather peaceful.

When the boat started moving, I opened my eyes and was pleasantly surprised to see my surfer friend standing on the other side of the entryway. I nodded at him and said something like, "Thanks for your help." He asked me if I ever made it out to that wave to practice surfing, and I told him I didn't get the chance. "Next time," he said. We had to speak loudly because the engines were revving up to full throttle. He looked at the full cabin and then he looked at me. "Claustrophobic?" he asked. I shook my head. "No," I said, "I'm just more comfortable right here." He nodded a hearty yes, and that was pretty much the end of our conversation. We enjoyed the breeze and the gentle bumping of the boat on the light chop and (for me, at least) the satisfaction of surviving my lap around Bali.

It hadn't been a full forty days and forty nights, but I was not too far from it. Later that afternoon I would even check into the same hotel in Seminyak where I had spent my first night. I was physically wiped out, so it felt like I'd done the full forty and forty. I was also emotionally wiped out. I don't like thinking about it, but I was sad pretty much all the time on this trip (even when I was happy). Sometimes—like when I was talking to the old surfer or snorkeling the wreck—the sadness moved toward the stern of my mind. But like the tide that kept pushing those boats toward shore, it would always return, and I'd get tripped up on the ropes of loss, of missing, of longing, of grief. I sat on the edge of a bed in Seminyak, held my head in my hands, and cried. And I sat on the edge of a bed in Pemuteran and cried. And in Tulamben, where that rat was lurking in some unseen corner. And so on. I was hoping that something was being exorcized, and that by the time I made it to Borneo and the orangutans, the worst would be behind me.

———

ON MY SECOND AFTERNOON in Seminyak, I got sick. I woke from a nap with a fever headache, and I was immediately nauseated. I could tell right away that it was going to be a bad one . . . it was going to make what happened in Tulamben look like kid's stuff. It started about fifteen minutes later, vomiting and vomiting and vomiting, and it went on for many endless-seeming hours.

Usually, during these traveler's illness episodes, there is some respite between bouts of throwing up, a relative calm between the waves. But this one was different. There was no reprieve. It was all tsunami. And later that night, when I finally did fall asleep, I had Möbius-strip fever dreams, and I felt as sick when I was asleep as I did when I was awake. I didn't feel any better the next day or the day after that, which was when I was scheduled to fly to Borneo.

I pushed my air and hotel reservations back a day. Then I spent a third day trying to recover, but I made little progress.

When I awoke the following morning, I did feel a little better. I turned to my enormous duffel to get his two cents on the matter, but he was silent, so I packed him up and called the front desk to let them know I would be checking out and asked them to arrange transportation to the airport. Then I hoisted my ginormous duffel on my shoulder and headed to the lobby, where I slumped on a couch until a cab arrived to take me to the airport.

I don't know if my driver could tell that I wasn't feeling well, but he was a fantastic driver. He didn't risk our lives swerving around cars, and he didn't use his horn to get the stupid motorbikers out of the way. And his cab didn't reek of petrol.

The airport was just a few miles away, but it took forever to get there. I was feeling so bad that I kept thinking that at any moment I was going to have to ask the driver to pull over.

But I made it to the airport without incident, and that was a relief because I figured the car ride was going to be the worst part of my travels. I checked in at the international terminal, and here things get fuzzy. Did I check my bag? Or was Bali one of the airports where you check your bag right at the gate? Did I have to go through immigration and get my passport stamped?

I can't remember now, because on that day I was a zombie. I know I somehow dragged myself to my gate—at the far end of the airport—well in advance of my departure time. I took a seat and closed my eyes, taking deliberate, steady breaths, and it was in that moment between sleep and wakefulness that I decided with sudden urgency it was time to abort.

This part is also fuzzy. Maybe I used my own phone to call for help, or maybe there was an airport phone on the wall near me? I called the airline and told them my predicament, that I had checked in for my flight but was too sick to take it, that I had technically exited the country and my visa was about to expire and I had to retrieve my bag if I had indeed checked it. They told me to wait where I was and someone would come find me.

About twenty minutes later, a small Balinese woman in a uniform approached me. "Are you Brian?" she asked. And I said, "Yes." I presume some form of desperation dripped off that word because this woman really took me under her wing. She got on her walkie-talkie and spoke to some people and then she asked me to follow her so she could escort me out of the airport.

But technically I wasn't really leaving the airport, because fortunately the Bali airport has a hotel right inside it. The airport agent walked me through the expansive terminal while I apologized again and again for having to walk so slowly. I still felt sick, but I also felt a twinge of relief. I didn't have to get on a plane (to Singapore) and then another plane (to Kota Kinabalu), and I didn't have to worry about getting stuck in Borneo with some kind of medical emergency. Plus, a bed was now mere minutes away, and I fantasized about the many hours I would soon be spending in a completely horizontal position.

Just outside the hotel entrance was the smallest airport-security checkpoint I've ever seen. I thanked the agent profusely, and though I knew she would find it rude, I tried to offer a tip. "Please," I said. "Let me do something for you." She declined, and I said, "But you've helped me so much." I was holding out some rupiah. "You can buy yourself a beer or dinner or something." But she still said no. She seemed like an angel to me, and I'll never forget her.

At the front desk the immaculately dressed, immaculately groomed, formal-speaking gentleman asked me how many nights I would be staying. I told him about my predicament and asked if it would be okay if I just reserved for one night, and then tomorrow morning, if necessary, could I add another? He said, "We can't predict whether rooms will be available or not." So I booked the room for two nights.

He then offered to call a doctor for me. "He's in Denpasar," he said, "but he can be here within the hour." I told him thanks, but no, I was just recovering from a traveler's illness and merely needed some rest. He gave me my key, and five minutes later I was sound asleep in a clean, well-appointed room.

———

THIS MORNING I woke up early and couldn't fall back to sleep. It was still dark and I had eleven sleeping birds I didn't want to disturb in my living room, so I sat up in bed and found myself telling the next part of the story in my head, remembering each sentence because this may be the last story I ever tell. And as I did, it made me feel sicker and sicker. This is the downside of reliving the past.

So I started thinking about Two-Step instead and remembered the first time I saw him pecking around the yard with a lady bird (V. hadn't appeared yet). I was eager for him to get to experience some normal bird life, but he was so vulnerable that first year I feared he wouldn't get the chance. Mostly what I wanted was for him to find a partner and fall in bird-love. Does a pigeon feel joy and meaning when he finds his mate? It's hard to say, of course, but I know from experience that my pigeons never look more at peace than when they are in the nest with their partners. (And I have witnessed firsthand the duress they go through when they are forced apart.)

That day, seeing Two-Step with a lady bird for the first time made me positively giddy. As the couple pecked their way across the yard, the distance between them sometimes shrank and sometimes grew. If she got too far from Two-Step, I felt myself willing him to go to her. In my mind I would be yelling at him, "You fool! What are you doing?! She's going to leave!"

And she did leave. One moment she was pecking, the next she was taking to the skies, and when I looked at Two-Step, he wasn't even looking at her. I guess he had decided to let her go. Or maybe he didn't know what he was supposed to do. I was positively crushed when she flew off. Two-Step, however, seemed unfazed. When I stepped onto the porch, he promptly flew to my head. I guess I was his partner, and he wanted to be near me. But he didn't know what he wanted.

Months later, when Two-Step met V., they were thick as thieves from the word go. I guess he knew what he wanted after all.

––––––––––

TWO-STEP HAS NOW REACHED the age that an average wild pigeon lives to. (He is two and a half.) He has had a pretty remarkable life, I think, one filled with adventures and constant care and (I hope) an enduring sense of safety. But three summers and three winters for him is not enough for me, no matter how good his life has been. I want him to have three more summers, three more winters.

And why stop there? Why can't he live another five years? That's a lot of life for a pigeon. And, hey, why not ten more years? Pigeons can live that long (and longer). I suspect this desire of mine for him to have more life is projection. But I also don't like thinking about his death. And I don't like thinking about being on this planet without him around.

I sometimes wonder about the things he would get to see if he lived another ten years. Maybe at some point in the distant future he would have a nest somewhere outdoors where in the middle of the night he would wake up and from his vantage see the sky shimmering green light—the aurora borealis! Or what about a solar eclipse? Will there be one of those in the next ten years? What would that be like for him? I have heard that birds freak out during total eclipses. I don't want Two-Step to be scared, but I wonder if the phenomenon of daytime darkness would give him a thrill. Do doors open for birds? Can a shiver run up a bird's spine?

———

THE FIRST TIME Two-Step flew with a flock was at the pigeon bridge. He was up on the beam, walking back and forth like a jail guard, and of course all the other birds were ignoring him. Suddenly, all the other pigeons took off, and this time Two-Step joined them. The beating of all those wings sounded like the leaves on aspen trees in a strong gust of wind. I was giddy that day, too, watching Two-Step soar with them. Maybe they sensed how miraculous they were, the beauty of their flight, and a door had opened for them as it had for me.

I think if Two-Step lives another ten years, he very well might outlive me. If I live that long, I will have outlived both my parents by far. I don't have the same excitement looking ahead at my next ten years as I do looking at Two-Step's. Limited as I am by my lack of capacity, blunted as I am by constant pain, it is easier to imagine thrills and door-openings in the enormous world of a small pigeon.

———

THE LOBBY AREA of the Bali airport hotel was polished and fancy and had little nooks with comfy couches and hangouts. The open dining room was big, and the tables at dinnertime were covered with luxurious white tablecloths. The buffets were ample and the food first-rate. The people who ran that hotel seemed determined to do everything they could to make you feel like you weren't in prison.

My first two days, I slept and visited the restaurant. Sometimes I felt normal and would want to eat, and sometimes I'd have low-grade nausea and the most I could do was pick at fresh fruit, rice, or a pancake.

Though I started to feel a buzzing body-wide ache in my muscles, I continued to exercise. I swam laps in the pool and visited the hotel's tiny gym and lifted weights and rode the stationary bike. Looking back, I know this was the last thing I should have done, but at the time I believed without question that my way to recovery was through exercise. And the paradox here was that I seemed to feel best *while* I was exercising. But at some point, later in the day, I'd get hit with yet another debilitating wave of illness.

When the third morning rolled around and I was scheduled to check out, I headed down to the lobby and asked the same gentleman behind the desk if I could stay another night. He looked at me quizzically, and then he turned to his computer and started typing. Then he turned back to me and said, "Sure. You can even stay in the same room."

I spent another day much like I'd spent the first two: swimming, lifting weights, trying to eat.

It shouldn't have been a surprise that when I woke up on the fourth morning, I still felt lousy. Again, I went down to the lobby and asked the same gentleman if I could add another night. Again he typed into his computer and again he said yes.

I don't think the workers at the Bali airport hotel were accustomed to guests staying four nights. So by that fourth day I think I had become a curiosity to them.

And then I added a fifth day.

———

AT TIMES DURING my airport-limbo life, I felt pretty close to normal, and at other times I felt pretty sick. But the balance was beginning to tip in my favor, so on the sixth day I decided to make my escape. Instead of Borneo, though, I decided my next stop would be Singapore, where I could get access to decent medical care.

I got some advice from my brother (who used to live in Singapore) about a good medical facility and I reserved a cheap (relatively, since Singapore is expensive) hotel nearby. Then I packed my massive duffel and began my Bali-airport navigation for the second time. This go-round was easier (because I felt better), but also harder (because I had overstayed my visa). The immigration officials escorted me into a back room where I explained my situation. "I really had no choice," I said. "Why didn't you extend your visa?" they asked. And I explained that navigating the streets of Denpasar to an immigration office in my condition would have killed me. I asked, "Can I just pay my fine and get out of your country?" and they stared at each other and finally said, "Okay." I think they wanted to teach me a lesson so that I'd be too scared to mess with them the next time I came to their country. Of course, none of us realized I would never be back.

My brother suspected I had giardia. He'd had it before and experienced similar come-and-go symptoms. He'd worked through it—with some discomfort—and had it resolved with a course of antibiotics that let him get back in no time to working sixty-hour weeks and training for triathlons. My brother has always been helpful, but this was the beginning of him suspecting he knew what was wrong with me, even though what was wrong with me was not what he thought.

Giardia is widespread in Montana. The cows grazing at high elevation poop in the water, and the tiny parasites travel downstream until some poor person floating on an inner tube accidentally swallows some of them. Despite all the swimming I had done in Montana—in the Big Blackfoot with my goggles, at Rock Creek on a hot fly-fishing day, at Fish Creek in a pool of turquoise water so cold I thought my heart was going to stop, at Flathead Lake where I jumped off the dock at nighttime with the woman I loved—I had never gotten giardia.

However, one time I went to my rheumatologist—about ten years before this trip to Asia—and she got very excited and maybe even proud because she thought she had discovered an answer to my mysterious early symptoms. Her tests revealed that I had a different protozoan living inside me.

My rheumatologist was a very attentive, caring doctor—at least at first. As time went by, and her old reliable techniques failed, one after the next, and I failed to show any improvement, her temperament began to change. She would lean very close to me and ask in a solemn voice, "How are you doing?" What this suggested to me is she had begun to think that my health problem was in my head. I mean, what other explanation could there possibly be? No imaging or tests came back positive. Toward the end of our time together, she seemed mostly annoyed when I showed up.

But that day she was thrilled about the creature she'd discovered living inside me. She said, "You have tested positive for something," and she handed me a piece of paper. The paper was a printout of an article about a small study that offered a possible explanation for my condition. (See how, in those early days, she went the extra mile for me?)

"Cryptosporidium," she said. What that meant was that at some point in recent weeks, months, or even years, I had swallowed the poop of some animal (or . . . and let's not think about this too long . . . another person) while swimming in a body of water. I blamed the long swims I took in the bathtub-hot Gulf during those summers I spent in Florida, looking after my mother. One of those summers in Florida I'd had a bout of come-and-go diarrhea, and though it was almost two full years prior to the day my rheumatologist handed me that piece of paper, it was possible the crypto had been with me the entire time.

Here, finally, was a possible explanation . . . and with it a possible cure for the early array of symptoms I had at the time. She put me on a course of antiprotozoal medications, and we waited. At night, as I lay in bed, I would close my eyes and imagine the restoration I was experiencing. Brand-new insides, for the rest of my life! I imagined one tiny crypto getting knocked off after the next. But nothing changed, pain-wise. After a month or so, I asked her if we should test again, to make sure the parasite was gone. I was hoping the meds *hadn't* worked, and the test would reveal the protozoans were still partying in my gut. My doc gave me a poop kit and a couple days later I returned with my specimen in a little brown paper bag. It felt like people were staring at me even though I knew the paper bag looked no different from the kind of packed lunch the healthy doctors and nurses and administrators were eating in the courtyard.

That test was the first time I wanted a result to be positive. A positive test would mean the cryptosporidium could still be the explanation for my burgeoning illness. I remember how disappointed my rheumatologist looked when she told me the test came back negative. I was "normal" again. According to her, there was no evidence anything was wrong with me.

BACK IN SINGAPORE, I was once again strolling down a street while holding a bag of my own poop. Collecting this specimen was almost the first thing I did when I landed there (after going for a swim in the hotel pool). At least this time the bag I'd gotten at the medical center was white. It made me feel I was doing something more scientific than scatological. After I handed it over, the doctor ordered all sorts of labs and instructed me to return in a couple of days. Even though I was stranded in Singapore, I was feeling a bit better, hopeful even, that whatever was wrong inside me would soon be found under a microscope and killed.

———

LATELY, MY DREAMS aren't as comforting as they were before. I don't know why. Maybe it's because of a new medication I'm taking.

At nighttime as I lie in bed, I try to reenact my ketamine infusions. I adopt the exact same position in my bed, I wear the same beanie L. made for me, I hold the same teddy bear L. gave me. And I deliberately try and remember the very specific moments I experienced with L. so as to cement them in my soon-to-be-dreaming mind. Some nights she visits me, and I am comforted. (Like last night, for instance, we'd decided to get married, but the day was getting away from us, and the preacher said, "Do you just want to wait until tomorrow?" And I shouted, I think out loud, "No!")

Sometimes not dreaming about L. makes me feel like I am supposed to stop loving her. I worry that my conscious mind is lagging behind my unconscious mind, and one day I will wake up so angry that I throw the beanie that she made me on the roof and give the teddy bear to Two-Step and V. to peck apart. People have told me that anger is good, that it could help me to move on, but I don't see the point.

When I don't have comforting dreams, the mornings are much harder. Exiting my bedroom and entering the rookery can be jolting. The birds who are still unaccustomed to my daily appearance start zipping around the room, and Two-Step responds with high-pitched warning noises. Pigeons are loud when they fly, in part because their wings are incredibly strong and make *thwopping* sounds and in part because the structure of their feathers causes them to whistle. An engineer could explain why having one smaller feather that vibrates among the rest causes this whistling noise. All I know is that the phenomenon is called "aeroelastic flutter." (Isn't it amazing we live in a world so full of miracles that we have come up with a term like "aeroelastic flutter" to describe something pigeons have been doing since forever?)

It is still dark outside, so it is not yet time to tend to the feeding and watering of the birds. I am on the couch, where I have started thinking and worrying about all the things I have to do.

If I were a genie, and I could blink my eyes and get nine things done all at once, this would be my list:

1. Take all the soiled bird sheets and towels and cage liners to the laundromat.
2. Put up my outdoor Christmas lights (a semblance of normalcy that the neighbors can also enjoy).
3. Clean out the rolling cage. (I'd have to gather the little baby in my hands to do so!)
4. Go to the cheap grocery store (for the easy-to-make foods).
5. Go to the expensive grocery store (for the fresh foods my doctor told me to eat).
6. Go to the Target grocery store (for foods my doctor told me not to eat).
7. Take my own pile of laundry to the laundromat. (This is hard. My days of separating are over; it all goes in one machine now.)
8. Go to the secondhand store and buy some little baskets (which, when lined with a pillow sham, the birds can build nests in).
9. Do a deep clean of the house, the kind they do after someone has been bloodily murdered there.

IN SINGAPORE, I sat across from my doctor and he gave me the results of my tests. "Normal," he said, and I asked, "What was normal?" and he said, "Everything was normal," and I asked, "Then why do I feel so bad?" and he said, "You don't look bad," and I said, "Right now I don't feel bad," and he said, "Maybe you had a bug and you're getting better," and I asked, "Is there anything I can do?" and he said, "Well, I guess I could give you an antibiotic."

Antibiotics have wreaked havoc on me in the past, so I declined. I also didn't believe his explanation for my condition. Yes, I felt better than I did in Bali, but I was still having come-and-go symptoms. I was hardly normal. But there was nothing else the medical center could do, so I retreated to my hotel.

The following morning, I still felt wonky. But it was my last day in Singapore, and I could hear a familiar voice—the tough guy, the adventurer, the international detective who was my father—urging me to "man up" and grab life by the tail.

Back then, I had a fairly negative attitude toward zoos. I felt bad for the wild animals that were constrained inside them. But the zoo in Singapore is considered one of the best in the world, so I decided to chance it. I walked to the train station, sipped on a Coke while I waited for the train, then rode it to the end of the line. I didn't feel great, but at least my nausea hadn't worsened. After getting off the train, I took a bus to the zoo.

In recent years, my attitude toward zoos has shifted. Perhaps that is because I now reside in a zoological habitat myself, and quite often when I open the kitchen door, the birds don't even want to go outside. Some of them will perch on *top* of the open door and peer into the yard. When I roll the big cage out to the porch and open its doors, the injured birds are not eager to venture out. They linger inside the cage, and sometimes they don't come out at all. Of course, these are pigeons, a formerly domesticated animal, so maybe they are not representative of all wild animals. But it does seem to me now that what animals mostly want is to feel safe and close to their loved ones. That's not too much to ask for in this world, is it?

I don't remember much of what I saw at the Singapore Zoo. I walked a lot. I kept thinking, "I shouldn't be doing this." There were elephants and sun bears and red river pigs.

And then I came upon the Fragile Forest biodome.

Something happened when I stepped into that spacious biodome. For a moment, it felt like I'd been transported to Jurassic Park. I became aware of an overwhelming feeling of serenity. The glass ceiling was almost fifty feet above the forest floor. An inviting serpentine path wound through a dense tropical rainforest. After all the crowds—on the train, on the bus, and everywhere else in the zoo—it was a relief to see how few people were inside the biodome. There were no screaming kids or squabbling couples, and the soaring ceilings made it feel like a church. While admiring some lush green plants, I noticed something moving underneath them, and when I got closer, I saw that it was a miniature deer. It was the smallest deer I have ever seen in my life, maybe ten inches tall, and it scampered off on its impossibly tiny hooves. This "mouse deer" is the smallest hoofed mammal in the world, but it was clearly "at large" in the Singapore biodome. I considered alerting a zookeeper, but then I saw another creature along the path. A tortoise, I think. Only then did I realize that the animals in the biodome were free to wander about. They were supposed to mix with the visitors. I felt the urge to find a shadowy recess on the forest floor where I could lie down and fall asleep with some furry (or feathery) creature at my side.

But then I looked up. And I instantly felt the same thrill I felt all those years ago when I was a little boy up past his bedtime chasing fireflies. High above me, large winged creatures were gliding from one end of the glass ceiling to the other, sometimes landing in the tall treetops. These were the creatures I had come to see. These were the animals I'd seen filling the sunset sky on my first trip to Asia (moments before I passed out cold). These were the flying foxes.

The bats looked much bigger in this space. And prehistoric. Their wingspans were enormous. I watched them for a while, then made my way along the path to a staircase, which I climbed, my legs feeling incredibly heavy, to a wooden bridge. When I stopped on the bridge to catch my breath, I was startled to see a large flying fox right beside me. We were eye to eye. He was hanging upside down, on a branch, using the fingers on his wings to grab juicy slices of oranges and watermelon that the zookeepers had put out. I stood on that bridge for a long time, watching that big-eyed, bighearted bat watching me as he enjoyed his meal.

I frequently dream about the Singapore biodome. One reason (I think) is because of the way the animals are allowed to commingle with the people (and vice versa). But I also think it is because I often talked with L. about turning one room of the house we bought together into a sort of natural history diorama. We wanted to feel like children gazing with awe into the jungle or rainforest that was growing in the middle of our home.

There were all sorts of exotic animals in the biodome. Frogs and sloths and insects that looked like they were designed by Picasso or a schizophrenic mathematician. And there were birds. Lots of birds. There were ducks and parrots and doves. And, as unlikely as it may sound, many of the birds were pigeons.

I FLEW FROM SINGAPORE to Kota Kinabalu, a bustling city on the northwest coast of the vast island of Borneo. My hotel there was tall enough for me to have a front-row seat to the thunderstorms that blew up over the ocean every night. I planned to spend a few days in KK (as it is called) and then take a short fight to Sandakan, a port city on Borneo's northeast coast, and then take a two-hour car ride to a river, and then board a boat for a long ride deep into the rainforest, where I'd get to see the orangutans before they become extinct. The shy, long-haired orangutans live in trees and sleep in nests (like birds), and they were the main reason I'd come to this part of the world.

My first morning in KK, I went a couple of blocks down the hill to the harbor and booked a tour for the following day to some small offshore islands, then I found some outdoor stores that carried the items my river guide said I would need for the journey up the river. I bought a dry bag, a coat that was as light-weight as could be while still being waterproof, and some leech socks, which are designed specifically to keep very small, very bite-y leeches from crawling up your legs and driving you insane and ruining your experience of the orangutans.

Dry season had passed, and that first night in KK it poured in torrents. I opened a bottle of beer and turned a chair to face the window of my hotel room so I could watch the magnificent storm. I felt like I had overcome the worst of my mystery illness and was excited about what awaited me. I changed into my bathing suit, grabbed my goggles, and took the elevator to the rooftop pool. I've always loved swimming laps in outdoor pools, but never more than when it is pouring rain. It's the same thing for me with skiing. A sunny bluebird day is a massive disappointment. I want it to be snowing so hard at the top of the mountain that you can't even see the contours of the slope. I want ice to freeze around the edge of my goggles and for my beard to turn into hair-popsicle. In short, I want to feel like I am up there fighting for my life.

The pool was empty, though the adjacent restaurant was humming, and the raindrops were so big and fat they made huge dimples on the surface of the pool. And the rain was loud, loud enough for me to have an excuse to ignore the security guard (who was approaching me), and dive into the pool, swimming underwater all the way to the other end. But when I came up for air, he started waving at me. I stopped and pushed the goggles to the top of my head. "You can't swim now," he said, pointing up at the sky. "Lightning." My swim came to a quick end, but it only took that one lap to make the memory of swimming in that rooftop pool last forever.

The tour I'd chosen was one that would take me and a handful of others on a tiny boat with a single outboard engine to a series of four specks of island off mainland Borneo. We arrived at the first island, by far the biggest of the four, before any of the other tour boats. Snorkeling was one of the attractions at that island, but I had come for a different reason: to hike a jungle-forest trail that wound its way up and down and around and through the island.

I must not have been very sick, because the hike was hot and long, and I felt fine the entire time. When I got back to the trailhead, I jumped into the ocean with my snorkeling gear, but there wasn't much to see. I felt like I had been scammed. Adding to the disappointment were the ropes floating in the water that marked the designated snorkeling spot and made it look like a community swimming hole you'd find at some shitty lake in the middle of nowhere.

Of course, I didn't know it at the time, but my life as an "adventurer" was ticking down to its final moments. I lounged in the sun on the dock, enjoyed the sense of calm that came with feeling "normal" again, and stared into the turquoise waters, waiting for my boat to arrive to take me to the second of the islands.

(If a friend had said, "This will be the last time you go abroad, and the only coral-reef fish you'll ever see for the rest of your life will be in an aquarium," I would have said, "You are nuts." I would have said that it simply wasn't conceivable. Then a more troubling thought would have crept into my mind. If that *were* to happen, would this person even want me in their life anymore? And, furthermore, what if I couldn't even make it to an aquarium?)

Buckbee & Fitzgerald

The second island was even worse than the first. There was a single large structure where maybe they sold some food and drinks, I can't remember, and there were tables, inside and out, and dozens of tourists eating their lunches in the shade of some trees. As on the first island, here, too, designated snorkeling areas were roped off. I asked one of the guides why they did that, and he said it was to keep people from getting hit by boats.

Despite its unexotic appearance, I broke out my snorkeling gear and gave it a go. Beneath the surface, in the water made murky by all the kicked-up sand, I could see plastic sandwich bags floating like Frankenstein jellyfish and people stepping on the corals. Other snorkelers kept bumping into me, and I couldn't believe this was Borneo, the distant land I had dreamed of, the romantic, teeming-with-wildlife paradise I thought would mark the end of my forty days and forty nights and put me on the other side of loss. I realized, of course, that this was not the best that Borneo had to offer, that I was on a beach just a few miles from the capital city, but it did not feel one bit like I had gotten away from "the things of man," and the sense of loss clung to me like the neon-colored water wings some of the kid-snorkelers were wearing.

Around the bend from the lunch crowd and the untamed snorkelers was an isolated stretch of beach, maybe a half mile long, maybe fifty feet wide, with a near-vertical wall of craggy rock on one side and the ocean on the other. I walked along the beach until I reached a dead end of ancient, weathered boulders.

The sand was soft and deep, the water clear and shallow, and it surprised me that only three people had abandoned the "snorkeling mall" a few hundred yards away and ventured this far. I guess I just don't understand people. (Maybe, in the grand scheme of things, as my mother used to say, I understand a pigeon more than I understand tourists.) (Maybe, in the grand scheme of things, I understand Two-Step more than the woman I loved.)

I spread my towel on the sand and got toasty warm, then went for a swim with my snorkel and mask. I was alone in the water—that part of the ocean belonged just to me—and as it turned out, the snorkeling was terrific, and the door opened one last time.

There weren't a lot of corals, but there were little underwater islands of life, and the shallows stretched far out into the ocean, so there was no shortage of places to explore. Even a small bit of coral offers an infinite universe—hover there and pay attention and you may be visited by the thought that some of these creatures have been around for a very long time.

When I got cold, I returned to my towel and warmed myself up. There was a young couple fifty or so feet away, taking photos. Their quiet voices and laughter drifted over to me when the wind was just right. To the other side, maybe thirty feet away, was a young woman sunbathing in a white bikini. I wanted to talk to her, but approaching a young woman on a near-deserted beach while you are both in bathing suits is pretty sketchy. When she walked to the edge of the water and let the tiny waves splash over her feet, I got up and walked to the edge, too. I didn't get too close to her, but I was close enough so that she knew I was there if she wanted to talk.

I think it is safe to say that by that point in my trip, loneliness was becoming an issue. I've always enjoyed loneliness (or used to) because I liked to think about what awaited me on the other side. Once upon a time, L. waited for me on the other side of loneliness, far from the karst cliffs of Thailand. And maybe that's why the woman on the beach reminded me of her. Maybe she reminded me of L. because she was beautiful. (Maybe she reminded me of L. because she acted like I didn't exist.) After a few minutes, she dove into the water and began swimming. When she came up, her long wet hair fanned across her back.

I got in the water, too, but I swam in the opposite direction. I explored the corals and fishes and when I got out of the water,

Buckbee & Fitzgerald

she was on her towel again. I don't know why, but she seemed like a happy person who wasn't weighed down by loss or loneliness. I was glad for her, and a little envious. She was younger and healthier than I was. She had everything in front of her.

I was supposed to meet my boat to go to the third island, but I blew it off. I liked where I was. The guide was probably frustrated and angry at me, since it's likely he had to walk around the crowd at the lunch spot calling out my name before giving up, but I didn't care.

I lay in the sun some more and went back in the water. Rinse, repeat. At some point I got out of the water and the woman in the white bikini was gone.

The picture-taking couple was gone, too, and I was all alone. But it was okay, because this kind of experience, woven with threads of peace and beauty, was exactly what I had signed up for.

I stayed on that beach until the crowd near the dock began to thin out, then I gathered up my stuff and found a boat driver who agreed to take me back to the harbor. He said he had one stop to make, to pick up some folks at another location, and maybe it was because he saw the end of his workday on the horizon, or maybe it was because of the gathering storm clouds, but we sped along as fast as the little boat would go, and we were bumping on the waves and the wind blew our hair and the ocean sprayed our faces. By the time the harbor was in sight, it was spitting rain, and by the time I got to my hotel, the sky had opened up.

———

WHEN I WAS SIXTEEN, my parents would stay up late on the weekends to make sure I met my curfew. I would greet them in the living room after a night out, offering up some small talk that I hoped would demonstrate I had not been drinking. After a few minutes I'd say good night and rush off to bed.

On one of those nights my father entered my room just before I fell asleep. I was sure he knew I'd had a few beers and some sort of lecture or punishment was imminent.

"Come on downstairs," he said.

I put on my best fake-sleep voice and said, "I'm sleeping."

"Come down," he insisted, "there's a storm coming in."

So I followed him out to the front porch. My father loved storms. We both did. For many years before I became an angry teenager, my father and I would sit together on the porch and watch the darkening sky. Before I was taught division in school, he taught me to measure how far away the lightning was by counting the seconds between the flash and the thunder.

On this particular night we sat with our backs against the brick wall of our house, under the overhang where we could stay dry. "Look at that," he said when the lightning flashed. "Did you see that one?" As the thunder got louder and louder, I became more and more nervous, convinced he was getting ready to spring some sort of trap on me. He was, after all, a detective.

The storm was approaching. The air was so humid it was dripping. I could hear the neighbor's sprinkler making a ticking noise as it rotated and the splat when its spray hit the street.

The suspense was too much for me, so I finally turned to him. I was going to confess that, yes, I'd been drinking, but before the words came out, I suddenly realized something that put me at ease. My father was tipsy. He'd had a few drinks, too. He didn't want to punish me. He wanted to celebrate the beauty of the storm with me.

And it was a beautiful storm. We watched the lightning come, one streak after the next, followed by the rolling thunder.

ON MY LAST NIGHT in KK, I walked through the enormous fish market and did some good people-watching and some good food-watching. I decided not to eat, though, having heard some horror stories from other KK tourists (featuring scary words like "bacillus" and "clostridium" and "staphylococcus" and the old reliable "salmonella"). I wanted to be sure to be healthy for my trip the next day to Sandakan, the city at the edge of the orang-utan rainforest.

Usually you don't think much about it, but it takes a lot to transport your weight-losing body and weight-gaining duffel from one location to the next. You have to get out of bed, pack the giant bag, tote it down to the lobby, check out of your room, have a car called for you, ride to the airport, check in for your flight, then fly on your plane over nothing but thick rainforest, then get off the plane, retrieve your faithful companion (i.e., duffel), find a driver you won't feel is taking advantage of you, take a car to your new hotel, check in to your room, ride the elevator way up, and finally slip the duffel off your aching strap-indented shoulder, lock your valuables—passport, wallet, phone—in the safe, find a place—atop a bureau, under the mattress—to hide your laptop, change into your bathing suit, grab your goggles, and take the elevator up to the rooftop pool.

In Sandakan, after accomplishing all that, I was tired, but I didn't feel too bad. Still, the pool looked intimidating. I thought maybe it was because I hadn't eaten anything since breakfast, so I went into the adjacent mini-restaurant to get something. They were closed until dinner, but I asked a worker who was meander-ing through if there was something, anything, she could get for me. "Peanut noodles?" she asked, and I said, "Perfect."

I sat alone in the quiet restaurant and realized I actually wasn't feeling all that great. This was confirmed when the worker brought me the biggest plate of peanut noodles I'd ever seen in my life. I took a bite and realized I was in trouble. My appetite apparently had been left behind in KK. I flagged the worker and asked her to wrap up the food for me and headed back to my room. I put the noodles in my fridge and lay down on the bed.

I was scheduled to take a long boat ride deep into the rainforest the next day, where I would be isolated at a small guesthouse with a handful of other tourists who were all sharing the same bathroom. The food would be . . . safe to eat? Not safe? And no matter what happened there, in a couple days' time I'd have to take the long boat ride back.

So, yes, I began to freak out. I had already had freak-outs—in the Bali airport, for instance, and in the rat-room in Tulamben—but this was a new level of freak-out. I didn't know I was on the verge of entering the world with a whole new hardship, and that, as I moved through it, I would be forced to constantly ask myself, "What's wrong with you? Have you brought this on yourself? Why don't you just snap out of it?"

———

AM I TOO TIRED to talk to you about Sandakan today? (Are you too tired to listen?) Should we just sit on my couch and watch the birds and look at the Christmas lights and count the bird ornaments on the Christmas tree? Or should we get back to my hotel room, where I jumped on my computer and canceled my trip into the rainforest? The orangutans would have to wait. Even though my last-minute cancellation didn't just cost me my deposit but the entire expense of the tour, I didn't mind. A big-time, major-league meltdown was about to hit, and all I wanted to do was get the hell out of there. And I didn't just mean get out of Sandakan, and I didn't just mean get out of Borneo. I meant it was time to get home.

I looked at flights out of Sandakan—there were multiple flights every day—but at that moment I was in no condition to get on a plane or make even the most minute of decisions. I fell asleep in a curled-up ball on top of the covers.

Buckbee & Fitzgerald

When I woke up in the early evening, I had a fever.

But the fever wasn't my biggest problem. I felt sick again, in that new way that had been recurring in recent weeks. But now the volume was turned way up, and I knew it wasn't possible to travel in such a condition. So I went back to sleep, and I passed the night unvisited by rats or bathroom sprints or Möbius-strip fever dreams.

When I woke up in the morning, I still felt horrible. I retrieved the sickeningly large mountain of peanut noodles from my refrigerator and tried to summon an appetite, but the only thing that arose was my nausea. The low-grade fever was back, and even thinking about lifting my gargantuan duffel made my legs feel like cracked glass. So I did what all great warriors do in crisis: I curled up in a ball (again) and went to sleep.

I woke up an hour later but still felt lousy and went back to sleep. Then I woke up again, an hour or so after that. My first thought was, "Hey, I feel a little better."

What unfolded next I can only attribute to God being on my side. I flipped open my laptop and checked the flight times out of Sandakan. There was a flight departing direct to the Kuala Lumpur airport in an hour. I got my credit card, purchased the ticket, called the front desk to arrange transport to the airport, and packed the few items I had taken out of my duffel back in the duffel. In ten minutes, I was out of the room. Five minutes later, I was in a car on the way to the airport. And twenty minutes later, I was in the small, crowded terminal, waiting for my flight . . . that had been delayed by a couple of hours. I found a seat near the back wall and slumped in it. Occasionally, I opened my eyes to look at the other passengers, none of whom seemed too bothered by the schedule change. Even though I wasn't moving, I was relieved to be on the move.

When I finally got to the airport, I had a choice: I could either make a break for home or get a taxi to drive me forty miles to a hotel near a premier medical center where I could stay until I could figure out what was wrong with me and get on the mend.

The shortest trip time to Missoula, door to door, including transportation to and from airports and waits between flights, was more than twenty-four hours, which, to me, in the state I was in, seemed like an eternity. Even so, I decided that if I didn't feel any worse, I'd buy my ticket the next morning and hop on a plane.

After I settled into my room, I went to the hotel's cozy little bar and ordered a beer and some sports-bar-type food to pick at. I wasn't feeling too much pain, and I even had a little appetite, and my spirits were buoyed (as my mother used to say) by the fact that, as intimidating as the upcoming travel would be, I would soon be home.

———

I AM IN THE MIDDLE of a severe crash right now. It's scary, because even though I haven't really done anything physical for the past few days, my legs are not strong enough to hold me up through even a short, hot shower.

I currently have twelve birds flying or walking around the house. Though I have tried to make them feel like wild birds, they are becoming more comfortable with me. I hope when spring comes and I release them, they will quickly learn to be afraid of creatures who look like me.

They have slowly begun to encroach on my turf. At one point last night, there were two on the spine of the couch behind me, one sitting in a cardboard box next to me, one on top of the tiny fake Christmas tree directly in front of me, and—because I have my legs kicked up on the coffee table—one standing on my toes and then walking up my leg. I must have looked like a character in a Disney cartoon. If I made a sudden move, or if I sneezed, they all would have taken flight and there would have been chaos and feathers everywhere. But I had no reason to move . . . I was like a statue in a park, covered in pigeons. I enjoyed examining the spread pink toes and the funny amble of the bird walking up my leg, coming so close I could see the flecks in the gold ring around his eye.

Whatever makes the birds happy makes me happy. I have such affection for these creatures. I am so glad they make me feel less alone. I am so glad to have this one purpose in my life (being their shepherd). I am understanding them more and more, so I can behave birdlike and, as a result, they don't have to feel so scared around me. Most days, I have more interaction with birds than I do with people. Except for the occasional hug or fist bump, I haven't been touched by another human being in a long, long time. But I am touched by the birds when they stand on my toes, or when I pick up the little babies to clean the cage, or when I give Two-Step a bath. Sometimes, while I am killing hour after hour here on the couch, in the recesses of my mind I find myself thinking, "I am becoming bird." Maybe sometime soon I'll start understanding what the birds around me are saying. Maybe I'll start each day making happy, pleasant *chukking* sounds to a partner I have somehow found, and later, when the sun is high, we will fly together and stand on the telephone wires, looking out over the treetops at the swells the green hills of Montana make.

MY ESCAPE from Kuala Lumpur was not to be.

I woke up in my prison-cell-like hotel room feeling lousy. I pulled up the airline website and found a flight that would take me home, queued it up, and sat on the edge of my bed with my credit card in my lap. All I had to do was press one button and I would be booked and ready to go. I came close. My finger hovered over the trackpad, but I couldn't pull the trigger. Not yet, at least. I decided to take a walk around the busy terminal instead and reevaluate how I felt when I got back to my room.

Again, more walking.

By the time I got back to my room, my legs were trembling. It was hard to stand up and I felt horrible.

I guess this is the time to talk about what I mean by feeling "horrible."

This is what I always tell a new doctor on my first visit.

First, I tell them to imagine a stereo, and it has a knob for pain. We all have one. When I had an accident biking through the purple field of blooming knapweed in the Rattlesnake Wilderness, I turned the dial to, say, a four. When I sprained my back while overextending my arm with the Windex bottle while cleaning the huge front window of the Chicago apartment where I lived, I turned the dial to six. That time in Alabama when the doctor scrubbed the built-up layers of scab off my knee with a medical instrument that looked like a grill brush? I turned the dial up to eight. (On that occasion, according to my nurse, the doctor said to her: "I can't believe that guy just let me do that to him.")

But the pain I had been feeling was not an eight, nor was it a nine or ten on that dial. And it was not an eleven, either. What I ask doctors to do is imagine that there is suddenly an *additional* knob on the stereo. The *quality* of pain I was feeling was so novel that, when compared to all my previous pain experiences, it couldn't be measured in the same way. No matter how intense that variety of pain was (and it would get a *lot* more intense over time), the uniqueness of it alone made the pain hard to bear.

The next thing I tell my doctor is that the pain makes me feel like I am being tortured. I always imagine at that point the docs think I am using the word "torture" as both metaphor and exaggeration. So I tell the doctor something like, "And I really mean 'torture.' I've had lots of pain in my life, including level 10 migraine, but I would never use the word 'torture' to describe any of those pain experiences."

At this point in our one-sided conversation, I simply say, "It feels like I am being drawn and quartered."

I assume that the image the doctor has is of a person whose four limbs are tied to four carts led by four separate horses pulling in four different directions. This common interpretation of "drawn and quartered" seemed to convey torture pretty well, even though from my teaching of medieval literature I know this practice wasn't as common as the other kind of "drawing and quartering," which was being "drawn" by horse to an execution site, where terrible things transpired, and then getting chopped up into four (or more) pieces (which also seemed to convey torture pretty well).

As an aside here, relevant in more ways than one, drawing and quartering in the Middle Ages was reserved for people who committed the most heinous crime possible: betrayal. In particular, betrayal (or treason) against the king. Dante seems more liberal with his ninth and final circle of hell when he talks about betrayal that extends beyond the king. I don't know how I stumbled upon this metaphor for describing my pain. Was my unconscious mind at work? I have committed one betrayal in my life, and it was a big one, involving tender words composed in Railay, Thailand, on a computer, while rain pelted the banana trees, to someone I was falling in love with half a world away from me who I was not supposed to be falling in love with. I'm not really a believer in karma, or cosmic justice, but every time I use the metaphor with a doctor, I remember my betrayal, and I have to wonder if I am that bad of a person.

At this point, if my elaborate description has failed to move the doc, I will veer in another direction and say, "It feels like I have been poisoned."

That seems like the simplest and most accurate way to describe the pain, because it is a sickening kind of pain.

But I also realize the doctors may have plenty of experience with people who have been *literally* poisoned, and I don't know what that feels like. I'm guessing how it feels depends on the type of poison you have consumed. So here is where I make my final pitch. It goes something like this: "It feels like every muscle in my body has its own stomach, and they are all nauseous at the same time."

At that point, the doctor, in a nonplussed kind of way, will say, "Well, hop up on the examination table and let's take a look." This is what you can expect when you have an "invisible" illness, like ME/CFS or fibromyalgia or Gulf War illness, or when you may be the first ME/CFS patient your doctor has ever seen.

When I returned to my room after my walk around the Kuala Lumpur airport terminal, I opened my laptop and made a reservation at the hotel near the medical center. Then I loaded up my colossal duffel and exited the terminal. I stepped foot in Malaysia proper, flagged a cab, and drove away from the airport, and I was too ashamed (and nauseated) to look back.

———

A NIGHTLY RITUAL has begun taking place on the stage of my coffee table, with two of my favorite birds as the actors. One of the birds is the "beautiful bastard" I talked about before, a juvenile now, with splashes of white feathers on his face and body and luminous white primary feathers on each wing.

The other bird in the play is the spraddle-legged bird, the one I tried to fix when he was a baby.

Their nightly performance starts around 9:00 PM, when they both land on the coffee table. They spend some time together during the day, but this is when they come closest to being partners. Pigeons "kiss" as a courting gesture, grabbing each other's beaks, and they will do this for a while, then one of them will squat way down low and the other will sidle up and gently peck at the back of its neck, as if grooming. Then they switch, and the groomer becomes the groomee. Mind you, this is all taking place inches from my feet, sometimes even in the scoop of the blanket between my legs.

The next part of the act is when the black-and-white-splashed pigeon settles as far down on his haunches as he can, wiggles his rear a little, and "presents" himself.

Of course, this is how I learned that the beautiful bastard is not a boy at all . . . he's a she! This fact complicates matters greatly. The mating of two pigeons requires a messy athleticism on the part of the male, as he must stand on top of the female, keep his balance even as she shifts her tail feathers so her cloaca is accessible, and then for about three seconds he flutters his wings to maintain his balance while performing his baby-making role.

My spraddle-legged bird tries very hard to accomplish this every night. Meanwhile, his girlfriend squats as low as she can and turns like a sundial so that he will know what she wants, positioning herself to make it as easy as possible on him, and this is all happening while yet another episode of a stupid and/or romantic "binge-worthy" show that I am watching to distract myself from the headache monster is playing on the TV behind them. When I watch my spraddle-legged pigeon, my heart breaks. I can see that he wants to do it, but with his disability, he just doesn't know how to pull it off. I can see him wishing he could be a healthy pigeon, realizing how simple this all would be if he was "normal." He pushes off with his bad leg, but it slides across the slick surface of the coffee table. On a good night he will manage to hop on top of her for a second, but with only the one good leg, he quickly falls off, and she is left unsatisfied once again, and in the background, some plagued-by-demons cop walks the perimeter of a bloody crime scene.

What the girl pigeon does at this point can make you miss love, if you have lost it in your life. She proceeds to teach him. She somehow signals for him to squat low, and then *she* stands on *his* back. But she doesn't flap her wings and doesn't close the gap between them—she just shows him that all he has to do is stand in place and maintain his balance. She wants him to succeed, and she is patient and gentle with him. She'll get off him and sidle up to him, and he'll try to get to his feet, and he'll slide across the slick table and use his good leg to move back and forth behind her, looking much like an uneasy painter examining a work in progress on an easel, but eventually they give up, and she flies off one way and he flies off another.

———

IN THE POLISHED stone-and-glass lobby of the sprawling Kuala Lumpur medical center, I was assigned a number. When my number was called, I headed over to the intake clerk—there were rows of them—who was waving me over. She politely asked me what I was there for, and I briefly explained my recent health woes. I can't recall the exact order of things, but I quickly found myself in the waiting room of a gastroenterologist.

The doctor examined me and ordered some tests, but he suspected I'd indeed picked up some sort of stomach bug and it would be best to start off with a course of a couple of antibiotics.

I hate being on antibiotics, but I liked this doctor's approach: kill it all. He wanted to eliminate every enemy inside me with extreme prejudice. He was like Patton.

I was put on two antibiotics—ciprofloxacin (aka "Cipro") and metronidazole. It is worth taking a moment here to talk about what I have subsequently learned about Cipro. Cipro is a medication that comes with a "black box warning." In some people, it doesn't just cause pain in tendons but can cause complete tendon rupture. In some people, it can cause, or exacerbate, central nervous system problems. You may get a headache, you may get a seizure, you may get paranoid, you may want to harm yourself. You may suffer dizziness or insomnia. You also may "develop the inability to walk." Metronidazole does not have a black box warning; it just slowly trims away the biome that you have been nurturing your whole life the way an old Japanese man in a karate movie nurtures a bonsai tree.

(This is not to say I am against antibiotics. They are, after all, "essential medication," and the two I was taking save millions of lives. I'm just trying to say that weird stuff can happen when we put weird stuff in our bodies.)

While I waited to feel better, I continued to go through the same ups and downs, and every afternoon I took a walk to the busy mall that was near my hotel. In the evenings, I ordered room service—the only thing that even remotely interested my appetite, for some reason, was spaghetti and meatballs, though I'd only eat a small portion of it. In the mornings, I'd head down to the atrium restaurant, but instead of ordering the breakfast buffet, I'd get a plate of fresh fruit and a freshly baked powdered jelly doughnut. After breakfast, I'd try to stay in the swing of things by going to the pool. But the pool area was a ghost town. Despite the shimmering cool-blue water, a spirit of desolation hung over the place. It certainly wasn't as lush as the pool area at the Bali airport. I tried to swim a few laps, hoping to get into the spirit of being an adventurous foreign tourist, but it didn't take. I just wanted the antibiotics to perform a miracle so I could go home.

The other day I heard the historian Jon Meacham talk about "pivot" days in history: December 7, 1941—Pearl Harbor—was one of them. Though I didn't know it at the time, I was about to hit my pivot day. On one side of the pivot, I had a mild-but-mostly-nondisruptive case of fibromyalgia or the like, and I was fully functional, fully in love, fully employed. On the other side of the pivot were the ruins of a once-great civilization.

That night in my hotel room, I took a downturn. This one, however, was worse than the preceding nights. Yes, I felt poisoned, and, yes, I felt like I was being drawn and quartered. But the poison was all skull-and-crossbones, and the quartering horses were flaming black steeds from the depths of hell. I hemmed and hawed (as my mother used to say) about what to do and finally chose to go for a walk. I decided I'd head in the direction of the medical center. If, at the halfway point, I felt a bit better, I would return to my hotel room. If, at the halfway point, I felt worse, I'd proceed to the ER.

I walked along the dark, lonely road. No cars drove by; no people were out. It was probably around 10:00 PM. In Montana, it was 7:00 AM. I was navigating the cracked sidewalk and had almost reached the halfway point when the oddest thing happened.

My legs stopped working.

The sensation is hard to explain. My legs felt shaky, stiff, and tingly. I could stand up on them, but trying to make them move required mental concentration, as if I were performing an act of telekinesis. It was the strangest moment of my life. To propel myself forward, I actually began picking my legs up by grabbing hold of each thigh and then pull-pushing them in front of me. There was an added sensation, up near the top of my legs, under my hip, that felt like some sort of perverse tickling. I looked around and wondered what I was going to do. I was half-paralyzed and I was turning into a statue. I'd be found in the same spot in the morning, maybe by some Malaysian housekeeper on her way to work at one of the nearby high-rise condos. She'd see a statue of a man on the sidewalk outside the arts and crafts center, maybe a pigeon (!) or two (!) standing on his head and shoulders, and she'd think, "Those artists have gone too far."

And now the entire thing—the weeks of being sick, the forty-days-and-forty-nights thing, the constant attempts to refresh myself by exercising—it all seemed ludicrous, and I began laughing.

What does it mean that my pivot point was marked by laughter? I have never been able to make sense of it. Was it a reflection of my true nature? Was it a reflection of my encroaching madness? Despite the ebullience (madness), I decided I was going to the emergency room. But how would I get there? Maybe, I thought, I should yell for help, and if someone came, I'd explain that my feet got stuck in drying cement.

I don't know how long I stood there. It was probably a minute or so, though it felt much longer, and then I began trying to move my legs forward again. They were so "frozen" they didn't work at first, but then they thawed out and slowly began to function, and after twenty or thirty steps, they had returned to life just enough so that I could walk—albeit at a very stiff-legged pace—toward the emergency room.

At the medical center, I checked in at the desk in the spacious waiting room and was told to take a seat. I said something like, "Okay, but there is something really wrong with me," and I was told, "You'll be called back soon."

There were only a few other people waiting—an older man to my left who was wearing a fedora and a young couple two rows in front of me. They looked like backpackers, the kind that were slumming it purely by choice. They didn't have an ounce of weariness nor the stink of the road on them. They were American, I think, or Canadian. The girl, who had streaked blonde hair as if she had just emerged from an expensive salon, was holding her right wrist in her left hand. She was whispering to her boyfriend, "Should we stay? I don't know if it's that bad. I can move it."

"It" was her thumb, and I could clearly see her moving it

without much trouble at all. She could have hitchhiked or won a thumb war or put it in a pie. It wasn't bruised or bleeding or swollen. "I think it's okay," she said. "It doesn't even hurt that much."

I remember wishing—willing, even—them to go away. I was beginning to feel an urgency to see the doctor, and if they left, that would mean I'd get called back that much sooner.

But they didn't leave, and they got called back so the doctor could diagnose her thumb problem. That they stayed made me a little angry, and so I got up and returned to the registration desk. I was getting more and more anxious to see the doctor, and I couldn't understand what the hell was taking so damn long. "You'll get called back shortly," the intake person said. And I returned to my seat. I bent over with my head in my hands and rocked back and forth, back and forth, until my name was called.

I was escorted into an examination "room," my vitals and such were taken by a nurse, and I was told the doctor would be right with me. "It's that thumb girl," I said. "She's taking up all his time."

My examination room had curtains on three sides, and the bed, for whatever reason, was in the very middle of the small space. This unexpected bit of feng shui would prove to be a lifesaver.

I sat on the edge of the bed, dangling my legs and eager as hell to see the doctor. The seconds seemed like hours, and I got up and began walking around the bed. My legs had a little bit of that frozen shakiness in them still, though not quite enough to turn me into a statue, and my impulse was to walk faster and faster. Again, I found myself laughing out loud, because I imagined myself as a lab rat in some kind of perverse experiment. Around and around the bed I went. Then I sat down, but I could only sit for a few seconds before I just had to get up and start walking again. Around and around I went. After a thousand or so laps, I slipped through the curtain and went to the nurse's station.

"How long?" I asked, and the nurse said, "The doctor will

be right with you," and I said, "What's wrong with that girl's thumb?" I didn't get an answer, but I found myself obsessed with her thumb, her stupid thumb, which was all that was standing between me and the doctor.

Back in my exam room, I resumed walking in circles. Again, I tried to sit, but it was impossible to stay still, so I walked and walked and walked, and sometime around my zillionth lap around the bed, I began to moan.

I'm not a moaner by nature. In fact, I can't think of a time in my life when I have really emitted a genuine moan. And I was embarrassed as hell because I knew that the patients in the adjacent exam areas—maybe even people who were having their limbs hacked off or were gushing blood—could hear me. I figured the nurses could hear me, too, but I didn't care. It felt *so good* to moan.

I kept walking my laps, letting out the occasional moan, though now they weren't as loud as the initial one. I reversed direction and walked around and around clockwise.

Finally, I went out to the nurse's station again and said, "I think there is something really wrong with me," and the nurse said, "The doctor will be right with you," and I mumbled something like, "How long does it take to saw off a blonde girl's thumb?"

When the doctor came in, I sat down on the bed and he started asking me questions. In a halting voice, I explained as best I could what was going on while rocking rhythmically back and forth. I assumed that he assumed I was on drugs. So I said, "I'm not on drugs."

The doctor was very calm, which was like a warm breeze on a cold day. He had the white coat and the stethoscope around his neck and the look and demeanor of a TV doctor. He gave me a quick examination and said, "I think I know what is wrong with you," and I said, "What's that?" and he said, "Have you ever had a panic attack?" and I said, "No," and he said, "Well it's not one of those, but that's the best way to describe it." He told me he would be right back and he returned almost immediately with a tiny paper cup that had some pills in it. "Take these," he said. "Benadryl."

He had such a great bedside manner—I really liked that guy—even though what he had given me was merely a pill I could buy some version of right over the counter in an American drugstore.

"What you have," he said, "is called 'akathisia.'" I asked him how he knew what I had wasn't a panic attack, and this was very important to me at the moment, because I was feeling ashamed that "it was all in my head," and not just this attack, but all of it, going weeks back. Maybe even years back! Maybe the seizures I had—even though I had them only when I was asleep—were brought on by something in my head. And maybe the passing out—even though it happened without any warning whatsoever—was in my head. When so many people doubt you, you doubt yourself, even though you know there is no reason to doubt.

"With a panic attack," the doctor said, "I look for five things." And then he told me what the five things were. I forget them now. I think it was rapid breathing, sweating, flushing, increased heart rate, and something else. "And you have none of those," he said.

By this point we'd been talking for several minutes, and he asked, "How are you feeling now?" And I said, "A little better." And he said, "I'll be back in a couple of minutes. Try and sit down."

When he returned, ten or fifteen minutes later, he asked how I was feeling. And I said, "I feel fine."

Ever since, when I hear the word "Benadryl," I find myself smiling, as if I am fondly remembering an old friend. Because not only did the Benadryl make me feel completely better, but the fact that it worked confirmed the diagnosis. I'd had an attack all right, but it wasn't panic, it was akathisia.

Akathisia is a not-so-understood phenomenon that is most

often brought on by the use of certain medications—usually antidepressants or antipsychotic drugs. Some medical conditions—like Parkinson's—can also cause akathisia.

But I wasn't on those kinds of meds and I didn't have any of those medical conditions. Furthermore, the akathisia I had was, compared to others, extreme. My attack went well beyond what most people feel when they have an akathisia episode. I know what I just described may not sound like such a horrible thing, but believe me, if you have never had it, it is a nightmare. The episode made me rethink my response to the restless leg syndrome commercials I'd seen on TV. Imagine having an itch that drives you mad, but it's not an itch, it's an itch's itch, and no matter how hard you scratch, the itch continues. Imagine you are witnessing yourself going insane in time-lapse motion. I guess if you have had a panic attack, you get the idea. Doctors worry about people who have chronic akathisia because it can cause them to start killing—themselves, others, *masses* of others. I heard someone refer to the attack I had as "chemical terror," and that, I think, sums it up pretty neatly.

———

I CAN'T RECALL NOW if it was because my akathisia attack was so unusual, or if there was some other reason, but the doctor wanted to keep me around for a while to keep an eye on me. I was led to another examination room, put in another hospital bed, and hooked up to wires and tubes. The holiday season was upon us, and in the giving spirit, I handed over more specimens, this time blood and urine. I reclined in the bed, so relieved the akathisia was gone that I didn't care about the low-grade pain and sickness I was feeling. I'd been in the exam room for about an hour when an orderly wandered through. He was taking out the trash or restocking supplies or doing some other routine task, but he apparently felt like chatting. "What are you in for?" he asked, and I said, "I had an akathisia attack," and he said, "Oh, you're *that* guy."

When he said it, his eyebrows kind of went up, and a look of recognition—and, daresay, excitement?—crossed his face. It appeared that I was an object of curiosity or conversation outside my curtained walls. "Do you know what's wrong with me?" I asked, and he said, "Oh, yeah, but the doctor will be in soon," and I said, "How soon?" and he said, "It's nothing to worry about."

So now—added to my sense of relief—was a sense of anticipation. Something had been discovered! (I *wasn't* crazy.) And I was about to learn what it was.

——

WHEN THE DOCTOR CAME IN, I waited for him to reveal my diagnosis. It felt like someone, maybe in a surgical gown, should have been sitting in the corner playing a drumroll. He said, "Your tests came back. You're positive for leptospirosis."

Leptospirosis! I had never heard this word before. Leptospirosis. Maybe it was a bug of some sort, or maybe it was a disease. That the name was heretofore unknown to me, and long, and Latin, thrilled me. I finally had something—something real! The name alone sounded powerful enough to wipe away my worries about how I had brought this condition upon myself, that some weakness of head or body or character (or all three) had kept me ill (and weak and pathetic) for so long.

The doctor explained leptospirosis to me: "So you're a traveler in Asia, and you're going from remote place to remote place, and these places don't have first-world hygiene, and in the kitchen of some restaurant the cases of soda are stacked atop one another, and one day some rat decides to hang out there, and then the next day you order one of those sodas and drink from the can, and then you get leptospirosis." That sounded like something that could easily have happened to me. "Essentially," the doc said, "you have rat urine disease."

Rat urine disease! Glamorous? No. But all things considered, I'd take it. Rat urine disease. I listened happily as he talked to me about rat urine disease. He said there were other ways to get it, but since I hadn't been working with domesticated animals in the Balinese farm country, and the pools I'd been swimming in were chlorinated, he was guessing rat. The incubation time can be as long as four weeks, and the illness can come and go for weeks on end. The symptoms were headaches and fever and nausea and body pain. He basically described the previous few weeks of my life.

Dogs can get leptospirosis, which may be the one reason you've heard of this disease before. The doctor told me it tends to be pretty harmless and is treated with . . . antibiotics. "Only rarely," he said, "can it lead to complications," and I said, "What complications?" and he said, "Liver failure or meningitis." I think I said something like, "But the liver can regenerate, right?" I knew this because I have always wished I had the resilience of the liver. And I'm sure he told me something about the liver, and then I asked, "And meningitis? Lots of people get that, how bad can that be?" And he said, "Oh, it can kill you."

If you have read other travel-accounts-gone-wrong, it is likely you have seen the photos that the afflicted take in their hospital beds. In fact, admission to a hospital because of some crazy illness or accident seems to be a rite of passage for the adventure traveler. It is so often used in literature that it is not only a trope but also is trite. That said, the first thing I did when the doctor left my room was take a picture of myself.

I think the reason I took that picture, however, was a little bit different from why other people take those pictures. When I am (or used to be) deep in the backcountry—after I've hiked ten miles and set up camp somewhere off the trail—I sometimes think it's possible that no one has ever been in that exact same spot. In the hospital bed, I had a similar thought. I wondered if anyone else in the history of leptospirosis diagnoses had ever been even half as happy with their diagnosis as I was. So, yes, I took that same overdone traveler-in-hospital-bed picture, but I took it because I was flat-out ecstatic.

What I felt in my post-akathisia state while leptosporidi swam through my veins was relief. If there was a physical, visible, testable manifestation of what was wrong with me, then I no longer had to worry that my illness was my own fault. Did I have rat urine disease? Yes, I had rat urine disease! I wanted to shout it from the rooftops. I wanted the whole world to know! That hard-to-spell Latin word was saving my life.

I no longer had to fret over how much I should walk or swim. I didn't have to worry about whether I should push myself or not anymore. I didn't have to force myself to travel in a sickened state to yet another remote place. All I had to worry about was meningitis killing me, and that felt like small peanuts (as my father used to say). I had started this trip wanting a forty-days-and-forty-nights kind of experience. I wanted to suffer in a cleansing way, in a way that would allow me to finally put down the giant duffel bag of loss once and for all. And now the time of worrying and pushing was over. Embedded in that Latin "leapt-to" word was evidence that I should not have pushed the way I did to begin with. In fact, my diagnosis was quite possibly proof that I was the opposite of the weak person, the skinny teen who disappointed my father and ran through the wooded suburbs in the middle of dark nights. Hey, guys—

(Dictation snafu! That out-of-place "hey, guys" was part of my dictation. I excitedly shouted those words because I was greeting a flock of pigeons that had just landed in my snowy yard.)

The pigeons are here for their daily meal, but I am particularly eager to see if the birds in "my" flock—the five house birds who spent the night outside—have returned. The black-and-white-splashed bird spent the night out; as did the bird who looks like Popcorn and was so sick when I found him I dug him a grave (but who has been fully healthy for weeks now); and the juvenile siblings, who have never spent a night out; and most worrisome, the bird with the broken wing (I have named him "One-Wing"), who can yet somehow fly (in the house at least) and likes to stand on the spine of the couch just by my right shoulder so we can stare curiously (longingly) at each other (but who might not fare so well soaring below the clouds in formation with a couple dozen other birds).

I just stopped my dictation and went out to check on the flock. None of my birds were in the flock. Not a single one. This is going to be a long day.

———

YESTERDAY, I USED what little energy I had to do some much-much-much-needed cleaning. I wore an N95 mask, but my beard is so long and unkempt I'm not sure it even works. I turned off the heat and opened the door to let fresh air circulate and give the birds a chance to go out and explore if they wanted. Nobody moved, not at first, but after about half an hour they all went outside, except for the baby, who left the cage for the first time just last week and was quite content to stay inside with me. I wasn't very worried, because in the past when I gave my other rescue pigeons the chance to go out, they tended to return to the porch sometime before dusk and hang around until I opened the door to let them in.

Two-Step and V. came back early in the afternoon. And the spraddle-legged bird shortly thereafter. In the late afternoon, I again turned off the heat and left the door open, but nobody else returned.

———

THE HOUSE WAS much quieter last night. And I suddenly felt afraid of an approaching confluence of events. I'm near the end of telling this story, and when spring comes, all the birds will leave the house for good. I'm going to have someone build an aviary on my porch, and it will be for the injured couple, the spraddle-legged bird, and One-Wing, if he comes back. The birds are on the verge of release.

My house is a lonely place without twelve birds flying around. Having six birds flying around isn't enough for me—it's not enough beauty or distraction or commotion. And zero birds? What happens to a person with zero birds?

I spent a lot of last night watching the spraddle-legged bird. He only stayed out a couple of hours, and he returned without his semi-partner. I wonder why he came back but his partner did not. Has he learned that his disability prevents him from living a safe life outside? And why did his partner not come back with him? Did she resent him for not wanting to stay out with her? Was she trying to teach him a lesson? He did look lonely last night, in his box all by himself, antsy. Maybe she can't accept him for what he lacks.

I just went outside and fed the flock. The birds from my menagerie still aren't here. Maybe they are holed up together somewhere, under some bridge or on some rooftop, and they are waiting for it to get lighter out before coming back home. (One great thing about having pigeons: you never have to worry about them getting lost.) I've turned the heat off again and my door is open. It is forty-four degrees outside and fifty degrees inside. I'm so cold my shoulders are frozen and my neck is aching, but I just want my birds back.

Before moving ahead, I have a report: the black-and-white-splashed pigeon, the spraddle-legged's partner, just returned. She immediately joined him in the box, and they groomed each other's necks, and he pushed off his bad leg so he could sidle up right beside her, and they are lying together in total peace. They look like they want for nothing.

MY CASE OF LEPTOSPIROSIS didn't seem too serious, so I'm not sure why the doctor admitted me to the hospital in Kuala Lumpur. Maybe it was because my overall health was poor, maybe it was because of the violence of the akathisia, or maybe he realized I really didn't have anywhere else better to be.

My room had more in common with a nice hotel room than a hospital room. There was comfortable furniture and a good view. Nurses came in from time to time to give me medication and check my vitals. I made calls to my brother and a couple of friends back in the States to let them know what was going on. I made sure not to make a big fuss out of the fact that it turned out I indeed had a "real" illness, but it felt good to be tossing fancy words at them that they had never heard before.

When my doctor made his rounds, I asked him if I could stop the other antibiotics, and he said that would be fine, and so that was good news. My brother, from his days living in Singapore, had an acquaintance in Kuala Lumpur who visited me at the hospital and made a point of asking the doctors a bunch of questions so that they knew there was someone advocating on my behalf and I wasn't a patient they could slack off on. He also did the yeoman's work of going to my hotel room and packing all my stuff in the Brobdingnagian duffel and checking me out of my last Asian hotel. During my stay in the hospital, he stopped by to visit a number of times. He had two young kids and a busy professional life and ran a Christian ministry for children, but he never made me feel like I was a burden. Simply put, he is a good man. And for that reason I want to be sure to include his name in this story. His name is Jimmy.

On that day, I found myself getting excited about the life that was waiting for me back home. I'd have hockey and my students and perhaps I was even ready to find someone new who wanted to open doors with me.

LAST WEEK, I went to the home resources center to see if I could find someone to help me build the aviary. In the yard were piles of lumber and stacks of secondhand bricks and ripped-out sinks that were strewn about like teeth punched out of some-one's mouth. The woman I approached not only said she knew of a builder who could do that kind of work, but also told me about how her ambition was to start a nonprofit that connects skilled laborers with disabled people like me. She immediately recognized the importance of this project and the difficulty I was facing in moving the birds out of their home.

She connected me with a native Floridian who recently relo-cated to Montana via Alaska. He is a handyman, an artist, and an animal lover, and he is approaching the project with metic-ulous care and a warm gravitas that to me evokes the spirit of a medieval cathedral architect.

The aviary will be made of recycled lumber and wire "cloth" (think raccoon-bite-proof mesh). He is designing it so that twenty square feet will be in the yard and twenty square feet will be on the porch. Having the pigeons so close to the house will make it easier for me than if they were moved out by the shed or to a far part of the yard. If I stretch my imagination, I can make myself believe that the aviary is merely an addition to my house and I am not moving the pigeons out at all. The shade from the overhang on the porch will keep the pigeons cool in the summer and protect them from hawks. The back of the aviary will be close enough to the house to share its radiating heat in the cold depths of winter.

After our initial meeting, the builder came back and showed me his sketchbook design. He explained that he was going to build the aviary in panels that could be easily disassembled and reassembled. When I asked him why, he said, "If you have to move it for some reason, you will be able to lift the panels yourself." I had barely mentioned my disability to him, but somehow he had taken note and built not only the birds' disabilities into the design, but also my own. He's attuned to people's suffering in a way I never was.

The aviary will have one door that I can walk through, so I can provide food and water for the birds, as well as two miniature doors built into that door—one up high for the pigeons that can fly and one down low for the pigeons that can't.

I have begun to think that what he plans on building will be nicer than my existing home. I am tempted to move myself into the aviary and leave the house to the birds. In the aviary, all my walls will be windows, and I will feel the breeze no matter where it comes from, and my ceiling will be a window, too, like in the fruit bats' biodome, and at night I will be able to trace the moon's slow march across the starlit sky.

———

THE NEXT DAY in Kuala Lumpur, my illness pattern returned. I felt sick in the morning, a little better in the afternoon, and worse in the evening. On his rounds my doctor asked, "Why haven't you eaten your breakfast?" and I said, "It made me feel sick to eat," and he said, "At least eat the protein."

But when my lunch came—I'd ordered poached salmon with potatoes and broccoli—I had a full appetite and enjoyed what was maybe the best meal on my whole trip.

But dinner was hard to stomach. And my bodily pain was worse than ever, the torture feeling, the drawing and quartering, and I counted the minutes until the nurse at the station brought me my medications—something for pain, something for nausea, something for sleep.

The next morning, still no appetite. I figured this would be the pattern until the antibiotics worked their magic. But when the doctor came by that day on his rounds, he had some devastating news. The kind of news that could wreck a person with my condition. I can't think of anything he could have said that would have made me feel worse. "It was a false positive," he said. "You don't have leptospirosis."

———

ALL MY MISSING BIRDS have returned, except for One-Wing, and I am afraid he got seriously hurt. Maybe he fell in the snow and struggled to free himself but ended up stuck, hungry, and freezing. I miss him visiting me on the couch with that look in his eye, the one that seemed to be saying, "Is it possible you could be my friend?" I'm worried he might be dead. Maybe in ordinary circumstances—like if I had a "normal" life and "normal" health—his loss wouldn't hurt so much, but right now it feels overwhelming. I would just like to see him once more. I'd like to know he is safe. I'd like to know he is exploring the world after his release, and maybe he doesn't feel so alone anymore.

I dreamed last night of circles of pigeon feathers, the telltale sign of hawk attacks. And in another dream—about what, I can't recall—I was disabled. I have never been sick in my dreams . . . until the past few weeks. Now, I seem to be sick and disabled in almost all of them. My dream life is not what it was. I used to get to feel like the old me in my dreams, but now I don't.

———

I HAVE BEEN TALKING about the same two things—my grief and my health—with my therapist over and over again, twice a week, sometimes more, for seven years. She must be so sick of me. Sometimes I apologize and tell her, "I really am trying to move on, I want you to know that." And she says, "I've never known anyone who has tried harder than you." (Of course, there are different ways of interpreting that.)

December is nearly over, and I'm reading what I dictated and trying to clean it up a little so my editor doesn't break up with me. While doing this polishing, I repeatedly close my eyes for momentary relief, and when I open them, they skip all over the "page," so I make a real mess of things. I am struggling to put my thoughts together. Carol Ann is going to the whip now. She senses the finish line. "Just a little more," she keeps saying. "We're almost there." I am so tired.

———

IN KUALA LUMPUR, this is how I responded to the news that I didn't have rat urine disease: "Are you sure?" I tried to hide the disappointment in my voice. I asked the doctor if he could run the test again. I said something like, "How do you know the first test wasn't the accurate one, and the second one wrong?" He just laughed. Something about the way the tests are done, unfortunately, made what I hoped for impossible.

———

THE NEXT DAY the doctor didn't know what to do with me. "We're not sure what to do with you," he said. "Your tests are all normal. What do you want us to do?"

I read between the lines loud and clear—he wanted me to discharge. But I wasn't going anywhere. What was I going to do?

Return to my fancy hotel and order spaghetti and meatballs for the rest of my life? And the pain that came and went was so sickeningly torturous that when I even thought about attempting to travel home, I felt sicker and more tortured.

They say if you have your health, you have everything. For me, not having rat disease meant I had nothing. Before my trip to Asia, I'd had my health (relatively speaking), but playing hockey (the game I loved) and teaching (the students I loved) and sitting at the bar in a nice restaurant and talking to strangers (who I might come to love) didn't make me feel like I had *everything*. When I look back now, I realize I should have felt more gratitude for what I did have. But at the time I was too aware of what I had lost. I was surrounded by ghosts, or ghost memories (or I was a ghost). Something ghostly was happening.

IT WAS IN my hospital bed in Kuala Lumpur that I felt the beginnings of nothingness. It's pitiful, but it's true. I was half convinced I was going to die in Asia, alone and soon, and I would never see L. again.

One thing I was definitely *not* going to do was leave the hospital. They could give the nurses crowbars and I still wasn't going to budge. This put my doctor in quite a conundrum because I think he was realizing something like, "Gee, if this guy doesn't leave now, we'll never get rid of him." I knew that behind the scenes my brother was talking to my doctor, but about the precise details he was a bit elusive. I felt like I was somehow being left out of the loop, and this only made me feel more pathetic. I felt like a child. A weak child. Was my doctor going to call the police and evict me? Is it normal for people to assert squatter's rights in a hospital room?

I JUST SAW ONE-WING. He showed up in the yard with some other pigeons. He looked healthy. I tried to coax him into the house, but when the other birds scattered, he went with them. His flying is still not great, but he seems to be doing okay.

———

I HAD A DEATH DREAM on night four of my stay in the hospital in Kuala Lumpur. In the dream I was happily floating in the current of a clear river, surrounded by red cliffs, beneath an intensely blue sky. As I floated around a bend, I suddenly realized I needed to get out of the water. Immediately. As I swirled past a large rock, a hand stretched toward me to help me out. I reached for the hand and just missed it. And in that instant, I plunged straight down—down, down, down—and I realized— no, I *experienced*—my imminent, inevitable death.

I have had lots of nightmares in my life. The worst were always about tornadoes or King Kong. But this was a new experience. It wasn't that I was scared of dying as much as I felt like I had a message to communicate before it was too late. As soon as I woke up, I knew that I had to stay alive long enough to somehow make it back home in case the woman I loved ever reached out to me. If she did, I would tell her three things: you're my best friend, you're the best friend I ever had, and I'll never love anyone as much as I've loved you. As last words, they seem as good as any others I might leave behind.

———

ONE DAY MY DOCTOR visited me on his daily rounds accompanied by another doctor. This was maybe my fifth or sixth day, it's hard to remember. My doctor introduced me to his colleague. She was engaged, intelligent, and had likely trained in the US, and she had some questions about how things were going for me. "How has your trip to Asia been?" "What was your akathisia like?" "Did you meet a lot of people on your travels?" "Why are you traveling alone?" In my naivete I dumbly and happily answered her questions. (It was nice to have some company.) But something was off. She sat down across from me and leaned forward as if she were really peering into me, like a hopeful lover fascinated by my every word, while my doctor was silent, standing behind her. When he finally talked, he said, "Dr. _____ is a psychiatrist."

And in that instant, everything clicked into place. It was obvious my doctor had concluded that my health problems were entirely psychological. He didn't believe I had a real disease. He thought my problem was all in my head.

To that end, he had enlisted the aid of a trained psychiatrist. He and she had clearly discussed their conclusion over the phone with my brother, and my brother—who was perhaps already predisposed to leaning toward authority when it came to my health and psychology—deferred to their opinion. And so they began conspiring together—devising a plan to get me out of their damn hospital and back to my home country. Their goal was to convince me that my problems were created in my head, there was no physical etiology of my pain/illness, and, if I really wanted to, I could go home.

Do you see Two-Step on the horizon now? Do you see how urgently he is going to be needed? Do you see why I have loved him so much? Do you see why I wanted everyone to meet him? Why I wanted you to see him take flight against the blue-blue sky and see how athletic (and majestic!) he is in flight, how all our time training together in the park has paid off, how he has learned not only to fly, but to fly with joy?

———

I FEIGNED INTEREST in what the psychiatrist was saying and nodded agreeably, while in the back of my head I tallied up my list of assets. When the doctors left, I got on the phone and called an old friend in Alabama. I told him what had transpired, and how stuck I now felt, and he said, without me even getting the chance to ask: "I'll come get you."

Twenty-four hours later, he was on the road. He drove from Tuscaloosa, Alabama, to Atlanta's Hartsfield Airport, where he boarded a fifteen-hour flight for Doha, Qatar. He had to linger in the Mideast until his connection to Singapore departed, and then he spent another twelve hours in the air. And, again, in Singapore, he waited for another flight, this one to Kuala Lumpur.

I had planned my escape from the hospital so that I would get to my friend's hotel near the airport at the same time he did. The psychiatrist made one last visit. She said she had some paperwork that might be useful for the airlines. The paperwork stated that I had a stress condition brought on by travel/illness/ etc., but it also stated that I had contracted leptospirosis. I still can't make sense out of why she did that, and at the time I didn't try. The truth is that by then I'd decided to take as many drugs as I could, and in my pharma-fog I tried to pretend that her diagnosis was the true one, that my problems were all in my head, and that I was in control over what would take place over the next forty-eight hours. It was delusion with intention, the only time I've turned to that tool in my entire life. I remember nodding at the psychiatrist, not to deceive her but to deceive myself. Yes, I had manufactured an illness. I'd been weak all along! I had mental problems. I was the kind of traveler (and person) who didn't deserve respect.

———

AT TIMES the trip home was easy; at times it was excruciatingly hard. I leaned on my friend to handle all the logistics. The letter from the psychiatrist caused all sorts of problems with airport officials when we showed it to them, probably because it stated I had contracted an infectious disease. For a brief while, we were convinced they weren't going to let us leave the country at all.

Odd problems arose when we were in the airport in Taiwan. I counted minutes; at times, seconds. I tried not to let on to my friend how miserable I was. I put on a brave face (as my mother used to say). And twenty-two hours later, we landed in the Seattle airport.

My friend had accomplished the task of nearly circumnavigating the world in forty-eight hours. (He would complete his lap two days later.) And at no point during his trip did he ever make me feel guilty, or weak, or that I was in his debt, or that he was aggravated by what was the biggest non-ask ask of my entire life, and for that I need to include his name in this story. (His name is Shrode.)

Finally back in the States, I felt euphoric. Of course, this was 8:00 PM Seattle time, so in Kuala Lumpur it was late morning, which was the typical time of day my pain and nausea would start its daily move "backwards." So I am sure part of my sudden bounce was just me being on my regular schedule. While we waited for our plane to Missoula, we sat at a restaurant, and I even sipped from a half-pint of beer. And then, in the freezing cold, we walked across the tarmac, boarded our prop plane, and headed home.

THE PERSON I HAVE BEEN trying to describe these past couple of months—the one who stumbled through Asia in 2018 with a broken heart—is not a person who was losing health and hope, not a person with a mysterious illness, not a person stuck alone in a hospital bed like so many pandemic victims would be, but a person who . . . simply needed a bird. And not just any kind of bird, but a pigeon, and not just any pigeon, but a particular kind of pigeon, a pigeon who could appear as if summoned from a well of need by a person who himself needed to be rescued by (whose life could be saved by) an injured, vulnerable animal who himself needed care, and through his need and nature could become a door-opener.

———

EARLY IN THE MOVIE *Joe Versus the Volcano*, Joe—an ashen-faced, bad-haircutted, monotone-speaking cog-in-the-machine worker—is diagnosed with what the doctor calls a "brain cloud." Joe is told the condition will kill him in a matter of months, but he won't experience pain. Joe responds, "But doc, I *never* feel good," and the doc says, "That's the ironic part," and he goes on to speculate that Joe's former occupation as a firefighter—and all the trauma that came with it—is responsible for making him feel so consistently bad. Then Tom Hanks's expression changes, and he suddenly appears excited (*happily* excited). "Brain cloud!" he says. "I *knew* it. I mean, I didn't know it, but I *knew* it." And from that point on, Joe is confident and energetic and never in the least bit ill.

I would like to have an ending for you like the one in *Joe Versus the Volcano*. I'd like to be transformed or, better yet, healed. I'd like to have some kind of life change like Joe has (he falls in love), and I wish I had a great, heroic, dramatic act to leave you with. (Joe jumps into the volcano.) But there is a simple truth: I don't.

It has been a year since I started telling this story, but I have not found an ending. One day is like the next, for me and for Two-Step. And I don't expect things will change much. The only change will be that all the pigeons will move out of the house, and I cannot describe how crushing their absence will be, because I have come to love them all, in ways that people don't usually love birds, or any wild animals, for that matter.

The day after I got back from Asia, I met the black monster for the first time. That migraine was one of the worst of the dozens (hundreds) I've had since I got home. I went through cycles of feeling awful for a week, then not so bad for a week. I saw all those doctors I mentioned, but none of them could help me. And why did I expect they would? After all, they are only doctors.

And then a couple of months later, in early February, during one of the not-so-bad weeks, I woke up and felt pretty good. I waited for the hit—body pain, nausea, headache, or migraine. (Maybe all four.) But none of them came. And by midafternoon, I felt "normal." In that moment, I had everything (i.e., I had my health). I expected that the next day I would have at least some pain or sickness, but again I felt normal. I felt good. And for the next forty-five days, more than six weeks, about a month and a half, more than a thousand hours, I didn't have a single moment of pain or sickness.

I remember like it was yesterday what those forty-five days were like. (They were like all the other days of my life before my trip to Asia.) I never worried about my health, not really, and I was totally convinced that whatever had happened was behind me. I asked my doctor when I could start exercising, and he said, "Any time you want," and the next day I slipped into the university lap pool, and I slipped beneath the surface, and I swam.

It was one of the best moments of my life.

I was home! I was in my element (and in L.'s). Though I had no contact with the woman I loved, she was a mere few blocks away. When I swam my laps to the deep end, eighteen steady strokes, I was swimming toward her. (But, of course, at the wall, I had to turn and swim away.)

And I was on campus! My former students were ambling all around me. I thought about how at that exact time in one year, I would be in the classroom with my new students and loving them like crazy as I tried to prove to them that looking at a text—and by "text," what I meant was the world—in a multitude of ways at the very same time can make them experience power and wonder.

But on March 19, 2019, the black monster returned. It was the worst migraine of my life. And when it passed, what remained was an intense (sometimes non-migrainous) headache. And that headache was still present when I finally was able to get in to see my neurologist ten days later.

With the fluorescent lights turned off, with the locale of the trash can identified, with the other lights dimmed, with my hat pulled down over my eyes, with my eyes closed more than not, I asked my doctor—because I couldn't believe it could be true—if a person could have a massive headache for ten days straight. And he said, "Yes," and I asked, "How long can it last?" and he said, "It can last forever."

/

THE HEADACHE THAT WAXES and wanes in intensity is like the moon L. loves so much, but it has never once gone away. When I look back at its inception, I can't believe that it was fourteen months before I found Two-Step (or he found me). When I think back on that time, I honestly don't understand how I lived without him. There was more pain then than there is now, and I remember all the questions from the doctors and therapists: "Have you thought about hurting yourself?" And I never knew how to answer that question. So I just told the truth: "Not in any *sudden* way." But I would add (because, as I mentioned before, I have the tendency to over-tell the truth), "I do think, however, there may be a time where it will be what is best for me."

I would always emphatically add that they had no need to worry, because if that moment ever came, I would take my time and include everyone, especially my doctors, in making any decisions.

I remember thinking, at the two-year mark, "I can handle this level of pain for another two years, I'll commit to that, but what happens then?"

It's scary to think that you may have to do that to yourself sometime. It is scary to think about the terror you might feel while doing it, the terror you might have as you sink into the depths of nothingness.

And because it is such an awful thought, the paradoxical result is you start thinking *more* about it, like when you're in your bed waiting to fall asleep with the company of your teddy bear on your chest, hoping you can come up with something that would limit the fear and terror. It becomes, in fact, a very necessary duty to think about it at length. And you start getting precise and creative, thinking about all the mechanics involved. "Could I buy a gun? What kind? I've never shot one before. Would I have to go to the shooting range and practice first? Should I vanish in the woods? If I took enough medications while deep in the wilderness, could I keep them down without throwing them up? Maybe I would have to take a lot of antiemetics? Would I have to research whether the antiemetic negated some of the strength of the medication? What if a wolf started to eat me while I was only half-dead? How could I do this so as not to waste the precious time of authorities—police and so forth—who might go looking for me?"

What I landed on was a scenario involving an inflatable boat off the shore of the Big Island of Hawaii over a great depth of water with a cinder block belted to my waist and two shots—the first to poke a hole in the boat so that it would eventually sink, and the second to poke a hole in me, and in the process tip me backwards so I could descend to my forever resting place in the opened-door world of the coral-fish seas, where I would be surrounded by the grown versions of the fish I saw in the tide pools with L. and the sound of whales telling other whales they miss them.

———

I NEVER WANTED TO DIE. God, I love this world. The only reason I ever thought about this stuff was because of pain. *Intense* pain. How long can a person live like that?

But as I said, my pain has gone down, for now. (I've been hesitant to talk about it, because I am terrified it won't last.) I am fortunate. Some people with chronic pain never get this much relief. They remain in agony, sometimes for decades, sometimes for their whole lives, and some of them never give in, and they are people who look like ordinary old grandmas or nice old geezers, but the reality is they are certainly the toughest motherfuckers I've ever met, and though I like to think I am not that weak, I doubt I could be that tough.

My capacity, however, has diminished. When I talk about capacity, I am talking about how many hours—or, more accurately, minutes—of activity I can tolerate without a severe backlash. And this seems to be the trade-off: I have less pain, but I also have much less capacity. If Two-Step were injured two blocks away, I would not be able to sprint to his rescue. If a good friend published a book, I would not be able to read it. (I haven't even read parts of my own book.) If one of my nieces got married, I wouldn't be able to attend her wedding. Some days I cannot even get out of bed because my legs are too weak to hold me upright. My baseline is inching down to the bottom of the chart. People often ask if I'm hopeful that medicine will make huge advances with this mysterious illness in the future, but as of now we seem to be no closer to a cure or a treatment than we were thirty years ago. We don't even know what causes it.

The irony of all this is that one prevailing theory suggests a connection between ME/CFS and a latent form of the Epstein-Barr virus, which makes me wonder if what I have began with the mononucleosis I got as a freshman in college, right after my very first kiss.

———

IN GRADUATE SCHOOL, more than fifteen years ago, I asked my mentor if he thought it was a problem that all my stories seemed to be about the same person in the same basic situation. (They always involved a guy who had suffered great loss and was struggling to regain his sense of joy and purpose. If this makes them sound somber and heavy, they weren't. My teachers said they were very funny.) My mentor cleared the papers off his desk and used a finger to trace an enormous imaginary circle across the wooden surface. When he was done, he asked me, "How many points are there in this circle?" I knew enough about math to answer. "An infinite number," I said. And then my mentor proceeded to trace a very, very small circle on the desk. "How many points are there in this circle?" he asked. "An infinite number," I said. He was quiet, letting the words sink in. And I understood the point he was making. Not only was there way more to the story that I'd been telling, but I'd never reach the end. The whole world exists in the tiniest of places. There is an infinite amount of space in a pigeonhole.

When I told my therapist that I'm too weak to do anything except water one small patch of lawn a day, she said, "Then that's your world now, your world is the lawn. Everything you need is right there." She wants me to believe that my lawn, with its green grass and flowering trees under the vast Montana sky, is an infinite universe.

MY CHILDHOOD HOME was surrounded by an infinite universe, too. Because it was in the floodplain of the Des Plaines River, this meant that sometimes pools of water would gather in the wooded areas behind our house. I explored the soggy, sparkling land, sometimes stopping to build a makeshift raft out of tree branches that I'd imagine floating on all around the neighborhood while looking for frogs and crayfish and any other creatures that might have joined the flood. Occasionally, my brother would join me and we'd visit a place we called "Deer Creek," a peaceful oasis that was slowly being surrounded by a growing number of corporate parks. Sure, we could hear trucks in the distance ripping up the interstate, but we were Lewis and Clark in the wilderness. We followed the paths the deer made, hoping to come across a fox or badger, but mostly what we found were rusting beer cans that older kids had left behind.

In those long-ago days I was most interested in the mysterious underwater worlds and the creatures they held. Maybe that's why I love L. so much, because she is a creature of water. Rivers, lakes, oceans, it didn't matter. Not being able to see into the depths made anything and everything possible.

I was the only one in my family with this interest, and I guess my mother understood this about me, because when I told her I wanted to take up fishing, I somehow convinced her to buy me a rod and reel and some tackle. No one else in my family fished or hunted or even went camping.

In the evenings and on weekends, I would get my rod and reel and ride my Schwinn Sting-Ray to one of the nearby corporate parks, which always had a sizable pond or lake. I had no idea how to fish. I would put a few kernels of canned corn on a hook, attach a bobber to the line, and toss it in the water. Sometimes I caught a bluegill or crappie or catfish. As much as I liked catching a fish, pulling the hook out was a problem, because it reminded me that this newfound interest of mine was causing pain.

Occasionally, my mother and I would row a rented boat out to the middle of Crystal Lake, and I'd fish while she leaned back in the bow and sunbathed in her bikini. We had a second rod and reel, but she never used it. I'd catch a fish, and we'd admire it, and then I'd carefully put it back. We spent hours drifting on the water together.

———

I WENT FISHING with my father only one time, and I'm fairly certain my mother made him do it. She may have thought a boy my age shouldn't be hanging out with his mother so much.

It was the middle of summer, when the days were long, and my father and I headed out after supper to a corporate park (the closest one possible) to catch sunfish or perch or the like. This is what had become of Deer Creek: the land had been leveled for a big parking lot, a shiny new building, and a man-made, chemically treated water feature.

My father did not want to put the worm on his hook, so I did it for him. He cast his line and then retreated ten or so feet to a rocky incline, where he sat down to watch his bobber. I stayed close to the water's edge, of course, hoping to catch a glimpse of some creature rising from the depths so that I could show it to my father. At one point I called him down to look at a giant goldfish that was swimming by. It was a fish I'd been trying to catch for at least two years. My father came down, but he didn't seem very impressed, and he retreated to his rocks, smoking cigarettes and watching his bobber. I watched his bobber, too, hoping for some action so he would understand why I'd been wasting so much time on this activity. Finally, it shook hard and disappeared, and I yelled at my father to reel it in. And he did reel it in, dutifully and without enthusiasm. He didn't even stand up. When the fish emerged from the lake, he just kept reeling, dragging it up over the rocks. The fish was flopping and gasping for breath when it reached his feet.

I don't know what I expected, but his catch did not excite him. I quickly slid the hook out of the fish's mouth and returned him to his home, and my father and I promptly packed up our gear, and that was the end of our fishing life together. Just because you yearn to go through a door with someone doesn't mean you can make it happen.

———

BUT IT WAS DIFFERENT with my mother. Six or seven years after my father died, my mother moved to the Lowcountry of South Carolina. She didn't have a history with the area, but she loved the landscape and (like me) she was comfortable moving to a place where she knew no other people. When I visited her, I would go fishing. While I'd be gathering my gear and getting bait from the freezer, she would be milling about, cleaning or preparing dinner, and there was always this easy harmony between us. When I'd come back from an expedition, I'd tell her about it. The brackish waters of those estuaries were filled with strange creatures—drums and rockfish and stripers, crabs, flounder. One day, in the very last vestiges of light, I reeled in something from that vast world below. At first I thought it was a snake. But when I set it on the ground, I realized it was the other serpentine creature, something I had never seen before in my life: an eel. Though I didn't yet have the right words for it, just like years and years later I wouldn't have words for what Two-Step looked like in flight, that was a door-opening moment for me, standing there in the windy salt air and the violet-blue dusk. (I guess they should have sent a poet for that one, too.) I know that part of the joy I was feeling came from knowing I would get to tell my mother about it.

Sometimes I would fish in the ocean outside the harbor where the mighty currents were moving in multiple directions. I would wade out into the water until it was up to my chest, tie a heavy sinker to the same lightweight Zebco rod/reel set my mother bought me twenty years earlier, and sling the line as far as I could. The currents would tug at it and I'd get knocked off my feet and try to dig my toes into the sandy bottom and soon the sun was so far set one could probably have called it nighttime. It certainly didn't matter if I caught anything—though I did sometimes, mostly catfish, which could sting like mad if you didn't handle them right, and baby sharks, with their unexpectedly rough skin.

When I returned from those fishing trips, my mother and I would eat dinner and talk and then we'd clean up. That was when she would begin *her* nightly ritual. She'd set out corn for the deer and carrots for any rabbits that might pass through and several paper plates filled with carefully arranged Nutter Butter cookies, which made those Lowcountry raccoons the happiest raccoons in the world.

My mother's house was surrounded by woods and the lush, wild things that grow in the fierce humidity of the Southern lowlands. After she put the food out, we'd sit on the rustic screened-in back porch and listen to all the nonhuman voices that sounded from the infinite world of darkness outside the faint glow of the house lights: the screech of an owl, the chirping of crickets, the tree frogs singing to their soulmates. And after she went to bed, I'd walk down to the beach and slip into the arms of the ocean, where I'd float on my back, wondering what was in the black depths beneath me while staring up at the billions of stars in the universe.

Buckbee & Fitzgerald

NEITHER OF MY PARENTS lived long enough to meet the woman I loved. I wish my father could have met L. God, would he have loved her. I think he would have looked at me differently if he had gotten the chance to see me with her. He would have had evidence that his skinny troubled teenager had come out okay. I think with L. and the boy I carried around a fierce don't-fuck-with-us devotion that he would have respected, and seeing those things would have made me seem different to him. I wish he could have met them both, and I wish my mom could have, too, and I also wish they could have met the bird I love. Sometimes I imagine a world in which all of us, the birds and the humans, gather on my lawn on a summer evening under that vast Montana sky, and my brother is there with his girls, too, and I stand on the grass watching them, trying not to lose sight of them for even a minute, before I head out to the store to fetch whatever they want and need.

Part 5

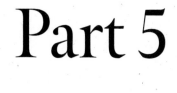

(JANUARY 2023)

IT IS JANUARY 5, NATIONAL BIRD DAY (AGAIN), AND THIS is the last of my dictations. Two-Step is healthy and lively and always in the company of his partner, V. As I mentioned earlier, pigeons in the wild usually live about two and a half to three years, and in a few months, Two-Step will turn three.

Two-Step's soft release was completed (for the most part) last spring, when I built the nesting box, attached it to the outside of my living room window, and Two-Step decided the box—like everything in the house—belonged to him.

Two-Step and V. liked the box, and they used it, but their home was still in my living room, where, on the high shelf in the corner, they had the surprisingly well-built nest I'd helped them construct. And since the front "door" of the box, their door to the world, was still covered, the box just seemed like part of the living room.

I went outside one warm day, stood on a stool, and removed the cloth that was covering the door on the front of the box. Two-Step was in the living room, and so I made tapping noises with my fingers to coax him into the box.

He didn't need much coaxing. He got in the box and promptly attacked my fingers, and we engaged in a back-and-forth duel as I slowly lured him through the door and out onto the diving-board entrance. Then I conceded the fight and dropped my arm, and only then did Two-Step look around and realize, "Hey, I'm outside!" He, of course, proceeded to stamp his feet on the diving board and turn in circles while making his "This is mine!" sound. And that is how he learned that the outside world and the inside world were connected, and he could move between them whenever he wanted.

I was glad my plan to release Two-Step was finally coming to fruition, but it was also hard because I knew how limited our time together was. In a few days, Two-Step would fly from his living room aerie into the box, and V. would join him, and I'd slide the window closed, and from that point on, Two-Step would never set foot in the house (his home!) again.

It was—and remains—a complicated event in my life. I'm guessing anyone who is a parent gets what I mean. Which is not to say I am comparing the magnitude of my soft release of a pigeon ("He's just a pigeon!") with your kids leaving home, but they do call it an "empty nest" for a reason.

But for me there was another layer of complexity, because what I was about to do to Two-Step I had already done once before. I did it to my mother, a couple of years after her early diagnosis of Alzheimer's.

When my mother was diagnosed, my brother and I moved her from the Lowcountry to Florida, where she could live in her own house in a small gated community where her sister also owned a house. Something about those first two years—the move, the meds, being near her sister, and maybe even the disease itself—made my mother feel wonderful. In some ways, I think they were maybe the happiest years of her life.

Fortunately, one of the first things my mother forgot was that she had a condition at all. But after two years, she couldn't take care of herself too well and needed to be moved to an assisted living facility. This, of course, meant having to move her out of the house she loved. We wanted to do it in such a way that she didn't even know she was moving.

My mother loved that house. It was on a tiny lake that had a resident alligator and was home to garfish and whatever other mysteries lived below, and at nighttime she could hear the chorus of frogs, and some evenings beneath the pinks and violets of the vast setting-sun sky, we watched endless clouds of dragonflies flying over from the nearby Everglades (looking very much like the streams of fruit bats I would see in the Andaman Sea years later and never get to tell her about).

I know what we did may sound cruel to some of you, but if you understand the nature of her illness, you might see what we did as an act of compassion. I wish I could take credit for the idea and execution, but that goes to my aunt and brother.

On that last night in her house, I said good night to my mother like it was the end of another ordinary, happy day, and tomorrow would just be another ordinary, happy day. But when I closed my guest room door, I felt as bad as I'd ever felt in my life.

The next morning we took my mother to breakfast at a place we called the "fancy restaurant" (it was actually the dining area of the assisted living facility). We talked about how amazing the food was, and the service, and my mother, who was always a trusting person and who was getting far along in her disease, went along with everything. She didn't realize we weren't really at a fancy restaurant, and when we told her we had a big surprise for her—and that surprise was a new condominium we had purchased for her!—she positively beamed.

The "condo," of course, was her new room at the assisted living facility. We told her we had bought new furniture for her and decorated the place and had even brought some of her things over and hung them on the walls and so forth.

My mother loved her "condo," and we walked around the grounds, taking in all the abundant nature—the white egrets, the fishing herons, the river otters playing on the muddy bank of a lake. As the minutes crawled by, we kept our happy faces on, and whenever my mother said something about "home," we redirected her thoughts to the new "condo," and then, when it got late, we turned to each other and said, "Maybe we should just stay here for the night? Wouldn't that be great?!"

And that's how my mother left her house, not knowing she would never step foot in it again.

———

WITH TWO-STEP, the key was the nest. Though they had no babies or eggs at the time, Two-Step and V. wanted to be near the nest, and so one day (whether I was ready or not, and I most definitely was not ready), I placed a chair under their living room nest, and while Two-Step watched, I slid a cookie sheet under it. This did not make Two-Step happy, and he landed on my arm and pecked and pecked, but it took me all of about ten seconds to get down from the chair and up on the coffee table so I could slide the nest through the open window into the far corner of the nesting box. I shook Two-Step off my arm and into the box and he stamped his feet and turned in circles. And then V. decided to join him in the box, and suddenly the moment was upon us.

I had started trying to release Two-Step six weeks after we found each other. We had gone for leisurely walks around the block, Two-Step hopping along picking up everything in his path that made him curious. We had gone to the softball fields, and I had "run" in the lush grass in my bare feet to coax him to chase me so that he would learn to fly. We had visited the pigeon bridge countless times, where Two-Step seemed to be most comfortable standing on top of my head. He was sick and vulnerable at a time when I had become sick and vulnerable. We were partners through the pandemic. We were friends, companions, family.

So now he had left the house and was in his box. I got down from the table, and though it felt like I was somehow committing grievous harm to both of us, I slowly, slowly slid the window shut, and then I closed the blinds.

A FEW HOURS LATER, when I opened the blinds to check on them, Two-Step had his beak pressed against the glass and was peering into the living room, looking right at me. This was his home, after all. And homing pigeons like to be home.

After Two-Step left the house, he didn't really seem to be interested in interacting with me all that much. But one gorgeous summer afternoon, a few months after he'd moved out, I was filling up the saucer-sled birdbath with the hose when I suddenly felt a familiar weight on my shoulder.

Two-Step had apparently decided he wanted to take a bath, and he wanted my help. He hopped from my shoulder onto the rim of the saucer and swished his beak back and forth in the water just as every pigeon does every time they step into a bath. Then his feet went in and his head dipped and he shook himself violently, the water spraying up all around us in a sparkling mist.

He did what he had always done when I gave him baths in the house. He turned broadside, lifted his wing, and looked at me. He held his wing like that until I played my familiar role. I put one hand on the other side of his body for support, feeling the weight of him in my hand, then splashed water again and again under his lifted wing. I rubbed the under-feathers, splashed more water, and rubbed again. And then he turned. He lifted the opposite wing, and we did the same thing maybe for the last time.

When he'd had enough, he hopped onto the rim of the red saucer sled and shook himself, drops of water going everywhere, and I got a whiff of that distinct post-bath pigeon smell on me, and then he flew over to a semi-shady spot under the lilac bush and settled into the unmown grass. I went in the house and started to close the door behind me, but at the last moment I changed my mind, and I left the door open.

Acknowledgments

Being limited to dictation means this book was never meant to be a "my" book but instead an "our" book. Actually, I had no intention of "writing" a book at all.

On January 5th, 2022, I blew the dust off my Facebook account and posted something about National Bird Day, sharing a bit about Two-Step and providing links to three different bird charities. That's when the people I call "The Facebook People" stepped in.

If not for their outpouring of kindness and encouragement (which I will forever be humbled by) I would have stopped there.

"The Facebook People"—friends and former students and people I cared for but had not heard from since the previous century—encouraged me to publish my early dictations, which amounted to a hearty essay. This is where Carol Ann Fitzgerald enters. A former editor of *The Sun* magazine and someone I had never spoken to, she said, "Forget the essay, let's make it a book." In my state of health, what she was suggesting sounded like an impossibility.

It is testament to how much I value her that I will respect her wishes and not go on and on about her here. She is the curator of my larger story, she kept me going, and she is the miracle worker who shaped chunks of dictation into a book.

But Carol Ann did even more, because she led us to a wonderful human being who happens to be a literary agent. His name is Farley Chase.

Not only did Farley contribute to the making of the book itself, and not only is his ethos of empathy and decency infused throughout the book and the process of helping the book find its way into the world, but he also led us to this force known as Tin House. We had other options, but will never regret choosing a group of self-sacrificing people who are true defenders of the written word. They made our book better, and they have brought it to you. Also, they're just really fun.

Along the way we received a lot of help from three talents and sharers of the ethos—Jenny Greil, Laura Munson, and Renée Zuckerbrot.

Of course, it all comes back to Two-Step, who would not have been possible if not for the love of creatures that my mother instilled in me, and the creatures I have been so lucky to spend time with along the way, whether they be bats or whales, dogs or fish, people or pigeons.